Parathyroid Glands in Chronic Kidney Disease

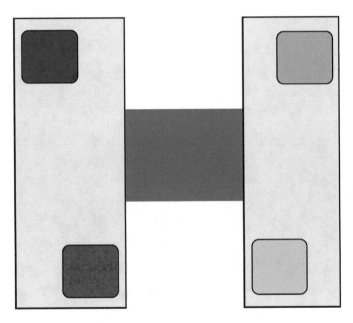

The Parathyroid Glands—in the manner of Pieter Cornelis Mondriaan (1872–1944)

Adrian Covic · David Goldsmith ·
Pablo A. Ureña Torres
Editors

Parathyroid Glands in Chronic Kidney Disease

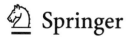 Springer

Editors
Adrian Covic
Internal Medicine - Nephrology
Grigore T. Popa University of Medicine
and Pharmacy
Iaşi, Romania

David Goldsmith
Renal Unit
Guy's and St Thomas' NHS Foundation
Hospital
London, UK

Pablo A. Ureña Torres
Nephrology-Dialysis Service
AURA Nord Saint Ouen
Saint Ouen, France

ISBN 978-3-030-43771-8   ISBN 978-3-030-43769-5   (eBook)
https://doi.org/10.1007/978-3-030-43769-5

This Springer imprint is published by the registered company Springer Nature Switzerland AG
The registered company address is: Gewerbestrasse 11, 6330 Cham, Switzerland

Contents

Parathyroid Glands in CKD: Anatomy, Histology, Physiology and Molecular Biology in CKD

Mario Cozzolino, Paola Monciino, Michela Frittoli, Francesco Perna, Eliana Fasulo, Roberta Casazza and Masafumi Fugakawa

Anatomy of Parathyroid Glands

The parathyroid glands develop from endodermal epithelial cells, in conjunction with the thymus. The superior parathyroid glands are derived from the fourth branchial pouch. These glands are closely associated with the lateral lobes of the thyroid and have a short line of embryologic descent [1]. The inferior parathyroid glands are derived from the third branchial pouch. These glands are closely associated with the thymus and have a longer line of embryologic descent, which leads to more variability in their anatomic position [1]. Inferior parathyroids can be found in the upper part of the neck as the carotid sheath and can also be found in the anterior mediastinum or even in the pericardium. However, the majority of inferior parathyroids are located near the inferior pole of the thyroid. The locations of ectopic parathyroid glands are related to the common origins of parathyroid, thyroid, and thymic tissue. The third branchial pouch contributes to thymus development as well as parathyroid and thyroid development. Both the third and fourth branchial pouches also contribute to thyroid development.

Normal parathyroid glands usually have a size of about $5 \times 4 \times 2$ millimeters and weigh 35–50 milligrams. Enlarged parathyroid glands can weigh between 50 milligrams and 20 grams, most often they are approximately 1 gram in weight

M. Cozzolino · P. Monciino · M. Frittoli · F. Perna · E. Fasulo · R. Casazza
Renal Division, Department of Health Sciences, ASST Santi Paolo e Carlo, University of Milan, Milan, Italy

M. Fugakawa
Division of Nephrology, Endocrinology, and Metabolism, Tokai University School of Medicine, Tokyo, Kanagawa 259-1193, Japan

M. Cozzolino (✉)
Renal Division and Laboratory of Experimental Nephrology, Dipartimento di Scienze della Salute, Università di Milano, Renal Division, S. Paolo Hospital, Via A. di Rudinì, 8, 20142 Milan, Italy
e-mail: mario.cozzolino@unimi.it

© Springer Nature Switzerland AG 2020
A. Covic et al. (eds.), *Parathyroid Glands in Chronic Kidney Disease*,
https://doi.org/10.1007/978-3-030-43769-5_1

and 1 centimeter in size. When normal in size, these are not usually identified on most imaging studies. In contrast, parathyroid adenomas and gland hyperplasia are larger and more readily identified on imaging studies.

The aspect of parathyroid glands can vary considerably [2, 3]. The color varies from light yellow to reddish-brown, while the shape is oval or spherical in most cases (83%), but can also be elongated (11%). Occasionally the glands are bi-lobated (5%) or multilobated (1%).

The majority (84%) of patients have four parathyroid glands, two superior and two inferior glands [2]. Only three glands are found in a very small number of patients (≤3%) and additional glands are found in 13% of patients [2]. The terms "superior" and "inferior" refers to the embryological origin of the gland, rather than the gland's location in the neck.

Parathyroids are located, in most cases, close to the posterior-lateral surface of the thyroid lobe; however, they can be found along the hyoid bone down to the superior mediastinum [4]. In some cases the parathyroid glands may be included in thyroid parenchima, being intra-thyroidal parathyroid glands [4, 5]. Although there is significant variability in the position of the glands, they are usually symmetric. The superior glands are symmetric in 80% of cases and inferior glands are symmetric 70% of the time [2].

Superior parathyroid glands The anatomic location of the superior parathyroid glands is relatively constant due to the close relationship between these glands and the thyroid gland. They arise from the fourth pharyngeal pouch and descend together with the lateral lobes of the thyroid to contact the thyroid capsule most commonly at the posterior edge of the middle third of the thyroid gland [6]. They lie under the thyroid superficial fascia, posterior to the recurrent laryngeal nerve and can be visualized with an accurate dissection of the thyroid capsule in this region. These glands may also reside inside the thyroid capsule, just superior and medial to the posterior tubercle of Zuckerkandl of the thyroid lobe. The recurrent laryngeal nerve is always anterior to the superior parathyroid gland.

On the basis of anatomic studies, the majority (80%) of normal superior glands are located about 1–2 cm above the junction of the recurrent laryngeal nerve and the inferior thyroid artery and within 1 cm of the entry point for the recurrent laryngeal nerve into the ligament of Berry and the cricoid cartilage [2]. Fewer than 1% are above upper pole of thyroid gland and only 1% along lower pharynx. None have been described at level of carotid bifurcation [7, 8].

Superior parathyroid glands can be undescended, or can be parapharyngeal, retropharyngeal, or retrotracheal within the middle cervical/mediastinal compartment. Enlarged parathyroid glands can travel straight down the tracheoesophageal groove or the retropharyngeal space into the chest.

Inferior parathyroid glands The inferior parathyroid glands have a more variable location due to their embryologic relationship to the thymus, as discussed before. They usually reside in the anterior mediastinal compartment, anterior to the recurrent laryngeal nerve. Fifty percent of the time, the inferior parathyroid glands are located along the lateral lower pole of the thyroid gland. Fifteen percent of the time, these glands are located 1 cm below the lower thyroid lobe. They can be located anywhere between the angle of the mandible and the upper mediastinum. They are most often found in the thyrothymic tract, or just inside the thyroid capsule on the inferior portion of the thyroid lobes. The incidence of intrathyroidal parathyroid tissue is quite low, approximately 2% [9].

Ectopic parathyroid glands Ectopic parathyroid glands occur because parathyroid tissue may co-locate with tissues that have a similar embryologic development. An ectopic parathyroid gland that fails to have complete migration during normal development is termed "undescended." The ectopic gland may be one of the four parathyroid glands or it may be a supernumerary gland. In a record of 102 patients with persistent or recurrent hyperparathyroidism, who required reoperation, ectopic glands were found in the paraesophageal position (28%), in the mediastinum (26%), intrathymic (24%), intrathyroidal (11%), in the carotid sheath (9%) and in a high cervical position (2%) [10]. These percentages will vary depending whether the ectopic gland is superior or inferior in origin.

Ectopic superior parathyroid glands Ectopic abnormal parathyroid glands in the middle mediastinum, anterior to the main-stem bronchi or in the aortopulmonary window, are considered to be the results of embryologic misplacement of a superior parathyroid gland [11]. It has been hypothesized that these glands develop there because the parathyroid primordium is divided or pushed laterally because of the passage of the carotid artery trunk during developmental events [12]. Such glands may often be supernumerary. Other reported rare locations of possible superior glands include sites within the carotid sheath [13, 14], the lateral triangle of the neck [15, 16], within the esophageal wall [17], or, less commonly than inferior parathyroid glands, intrathyroidal [14, 18].

Ectopic inferior parathyroid glands Undescended inferior glands, although relatively rare, are a well-established embryologic abnormality. The inferior parathyroid gland, which develops from the third branchial pouch, along with the major portion of the thymus, tends to move with the thymus anteriorly in its descent and usually arrests at the level of the inferior pole of the thyroid gland. A significant number (10–40%) descend further and are found in the thyrothymic tract or the upper thymic tongue. Fewer than 2% are pulled into the deep mediastinum at a lower level than the aortic arch. If an inferior gland fails to descend with the thymus, it may remain at its site of embryologic origin at or above the carotid bifurcation. Although anatomic studies suggest that this may occur in 1–2%, the incidence of an undescended abnormal inferior parathyroid gland is less than 1% in most clinical series of primary cervical explorations for hyperparathyroidism [19]. They may also be subcapsular, or completely intrathyroidal in 1% or may reside within or closely to the cervical or anterior mediastinal thymus.

Supernumerary parathyroid glands Supernumerary parathyroid glands occur in 2.5% to 15% of individuals [2, 20]. The majority of supernumerary glands are small, rudimentary, or divided. However, when enlarged, these additional glands may be responsible for persistent hyperparathyroidism after failed parathyroid exploration, especially in patients with secondary hyperparathyroidism or hyperparathyroidism associated with familial syndromes [2, 21, 22]. In a serie of 137 cases of persistent hyperparathyroidism after parathyroidectomy, supernumerary glands were found in 15% of cases [20]. They can range from 5 to 8 in number [3]. Supernumerary glands can reside anywhere from behind the thyroid down to and including within the thymus, representing the line of descent of thymic tissue during embryologic development. The most common location is within the thymus or in relation to the thyrothymic ligament (two thirds of cases) [3, 22]. The remaining supernumerary glands are usually found in the vicinity of the mid-thyroid lobe between two other glands.

Blood Supply

The arterial supply to both superior and inferior parathyroid glands is provided by the inferior thyroid artery in about 76–86% of cases [23]. Each parathyroid gland usually has its own end-artery. Most parathyroid glands have a single arterial supply (80%), some have a dual artery supply (15%), and a minority have multiple arterial supply (5%) [24]. The venous drainage of the parathyroid glands consists of the superior, middle, and inferior thyroid veins that drain into the internal jugular vein or the innominate vein.

During thyroid surgery, the surgeon should try to preserve all of the parathyroid glands in situ with adequate blood supply whenever possible. However, the blood supply may not be adequate following dissection of the thyroid gland, and the parathyroids are not always clearly identified. It can be difficult to make a reliable intraoperative determination of individual parathyroid function and patients may experience transient hypoparathyroidism despite having all four parathyroid glands preserved.

Superior parathyroid glands The superior parathyroid glands receive most of their blood supply from the inferior thyroid artery and are also supplied by branches of the superior thyroid artery in 15–20% of patients. A superior parathyroid gland that is supplied by the superior thyroid artery will usually be located in close proximity to the superior pole of the thyroid. A subcapsular dissection on the postero-lateral surface can bring to in the identification of parathyroid glands.

Inferior parathyroid glands The inferior parathyroid glands receive their end-arterial blood supply from the inferior thyroid artery. Therefore, gentle medial mobilization of the parathyroid rim from the thyroid capsule and preservation of the lateral arteriole going to the parathyroid gland is important for preserving functioning inferior parathyroid glands. Ligation of the branches of the inferior thyroid artery, close to the thyroid parenchyma and medial to the recurrent laryngeal nerve, may help preserve intact parathyroid vascularity.

Nerve Supply

The innervations of parathyroid glands is sympathetic, consisting of an extensive supply of nerves, derived either directly from the cervical, middle and superior sympathetic ganglia or from an intrafascial plexus located on the posterior lobar side.

It is important to note that these nerves are vasomotor, not secretomotor. Endocrine secretion of parathyroid hormone is controlled hormonally by variations in calcium levels: inhibited by its increase and stimulated by its fall.

Lymphatic Drainage

The lymphatic drainage of the parathyroid glands is carried out by numerous lymphatic vessels which tend to associate with those of the thyroid and thymus. Lymphatic vessels from the parathyroid glands drain into deep cervical lymph nodes and paratracheal lymph nodes.

Anatomy of Parathyroid Glands in ESRD

The overactivity of the parathyroid gland, known as secondary hyperparathyroidism, is a well known feature of chronic renal failure. It is an adaptive process characterized by an increase in the synthesis and secretion of parathyroid hormone (PTH), mainly due to some disturbances of calcium, phosphate, and vitamin D metabolism. The chronic increase in PTH production goes along with an increase in parathyroid gland size [25–27] due to cell proliferation that leads to an increase in cell number [26, 28].

Most ESRD patients with hyperparathyroidism (HPT) have four-gland enlargement. They can enlarge significantly, from 500 to 1000 mg per gland, remaining histologically hypercellular [29, 30]. However, some glands may descend into deep retroesophageal or paratracheal spaces, which makes them difficult to discern [31]. Patients with ESRD may also have enlargement of ectopic parathyroid rests in the cervical thymus [32]. Single or double adenomas are rarely seen in ESRD patients but have been reported in up to 24% of patients post renal transplantation [33].

Histology of Parathyroid Glands

Histologically the parathyroid glands are quite easily recognizable from the thyroid as they are organized in nests and cords of densely packed cells, in contrast with the follicular structure of the thyroid. Each gland is surrounded by a thin

Fig. 1 Normal parathyroid gland

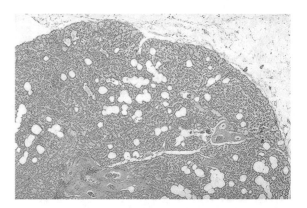

Fig. 2 A high power view of the parathyroid reveals two major cells types, the small chief cells characterized by rather scant, lightly-stained cytoplasm, and the much larger, eosinophilic oxyphil cells, which are often found in small clusters. The chief cells are responsible for the production of parathyroid hormone, while the function of the oxyphil cells is not known

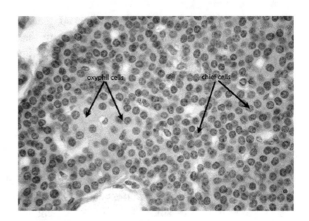

connective tissue capsule but it is not divided into lobules. The parathyroid cells are surrounded and supported by a reticular connective tissue framework, rich in adipocytes which increase in number after puberty, so that the cordonal structure is divided into clusters and cell nests (Fig. 1).

There are two main types of cells in the parathyroid gland: chief or principle cells and oxyphil cells (Fig. 2).

The chief cells are much more prevalent than the oxyphil cells. Their function is to synthesize and release parathyroid hormone (PTH). They are polygonal in shape with a round nucleus and they have a different structure depending on their functional stage: when inactive they contain fewer profiles of rough endoplasmatic reticulum (RER) and Golgi complex and they are filled with glycogen and cytoplasmic lipofuscin; when active they present a lot of RER, Golgi apparatus and secretory vesicles. These cells are small and pale eosinophilic staining. They appear dark when loaded with parathyroid hormone, and paler when the hormone has been secreted, or in their resting state. In adults about 80% of the cells are resting while in children more cells are active. Differently from the thyroid in which the activity of the adjacent cells is coordinated, in parathyroid glands the chief

Fig. 3 Chief cells: 6–8 microns, polygonal, central round nuclei, contain granules of parathyroid hormone (PTH); basic cell type, other cell types are due to differences in physiologic activity; 80% of chief cells have intracellular fat; Chief cell is most sensitive to changes in ionized calcium

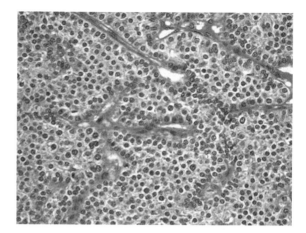

Fig. 4 Oxyphil cells: slightly larger than chief cell (12 microns), acidophilic cytoplasm due to mitochondria; no secretory granules; first appear at puberty as single cells, then pairs, then nodules at age 40

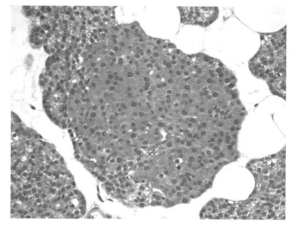

cells undergo cycles of activity and inactivity independently one from another, depending on calcium serum levels (Fig. 3).

The oxyphil cells are bigger and lighter in appearance than chief cells. They contain a small heterochromatic nucleus and their cytosol is eosinophilic, rich in mitochondria and glycogen. They appear in the parathyroid after puberty and increase in number with age. Their function is still unknown, however oxyphil cells have been shown to express parathyroid-relevant genes found in the chief cells and have the potential to produce additional autocrine/paracrine factors, such as parathyroid hormone-related protein (PTHrP) and calcitriol (Fig. 4).

Histology of Parathyroid Glands in ESRD

As already seen before, secondary hyperparathyroidism (HPTs) is an adaptive increase of the parathyroid parenchymal mass due to proliferation of chief cells and oxyphil cells in multiple parathyroid glands in the presence of a known stimulus for parathyroid hormone secretion. Chronic renal failure is a common cause of secondary hyperparathyroidism, which is one of the most serious complications in long-term haemodialysis patients [34]. The usual histopathological findings in this case is diffusive or nodular hyperplasia. In initial stages of chronic renal failure parathyroid cell proliferation appears to be diffusive and homogeneous, whereas nodular formations develop within enlarged parathyroid glands in advanced stages of renal failure, mostly in chronic dialysis patients with severe secondary hyperparathyroidism.

Compared with normal glands, parathyroid glands in ESRD patients have a preponderance of oxyphilic parathyroid cells, which is significantly more frequent in nodular hyperplasia, more fibrosis with a sclerosed architecture, and more dystrophic calcifications [29, 30]. Such shape and texture changes obscure a clear vascular pedicle, which makes shaping a parathyroid remnant more difficult.

Histopathological studies performed on patients who underwent parathyroidectomy for refractory hyperparathyroidism due to chronic renal failure showed asymmetric enlargement, nodularities and increased number of oxyphil cells. Nodular hyperplasia was the most frequent cause of refractory hyperparathyroidism in uraemic patients; moreover, it indicated more aggressive proliferation since in DNA analysis the relative number of scattered cells in the DNA synthesis phase was significantly greater in nodular than in diffuse hyperplasia. In addition, the calcium set point for the inhibition of PTH secretion was found to be higher in the cells from nodular hyperplasia than in the cells obtained from diffuse hyperplasia. Though there was no difference in expression of PTH mRNA in nodular and diffuse hyperplasia, these data suggest that nodular hyperplasia is more progressively hyperplastic, has more aggressive proliferative activities and show more abnormal regulation of PTH secretion. (Fig. 5).

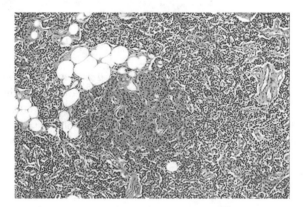

Fig. 5 In parathyroid hyperplasia, there is little or no adipose tissue, but any or all cell types normally found in a parathyroid gland are present. Note the pink oxyphil cells in the nodule seen here. This case shown here is "secondary hyperparathyroidism" with all parathyroid glands enlarged as a consequence of chronic renal failure with impaired phosphate excretion. The increased serum phosphate tends to drive serum calcium down, which in turn drives the parathyroids to secrete more parathormone

These studies also revealed that patients with higher parathyroid gland mass, longer duration of renal disease and haemodialysis treatment more frequently have nodular hyperplasia, and that oxyphil cells and acinar cell arrangements are marked features of this pattern of hyperplasia [35].

Physiology of the Parathyroid Glands

The main function of the parathyroid glands is to produce parathyroid hormone (PTH). PTH is one of three key hormones modulating calcium and phosphate homeostasis; being the other two calcitriol (1,25-dihydroxyvitamin D) and fibroblast growth factor 23 (FGF23).

PTH is synthesized as a 115-amino acid polypeptide called pre-pro-PTH, which is cleaved within parathyroid cells at the amino-terminal portion, first to pro-PTH (90 amino acids) and then to PTH (84 amino acids). The 84-amino acids form is the stored, secreted and biologically active hormone. The biosynthetic process is estimated to take less than one hour while the secretion by exocytosis takes place within seconds after induction of hypocalcemia. Once secreted, PTH is rapidly cleared from plasma through uptake mainly by the liver and kidney: 1–84 PTH is cleaved into active amino- and inactive carboxyl-terminal fragments that are then cleared by the kidney. Intact PTH has a plasma half-life of two to four minutes while the carboxyl-terminal fragments have half-lives that are 5–10 times greater.

PTH Functions

The primary function of PTH is to maintain the extracellular fluid calcium concentration within a narrow normal range. The hormone acts directly on bone and kidney and indirectly on the intestine through its effects on synthesis of 1,25 OH2D to increase serum calcium concentration; in turn, PTH production is closely regulated by the concentration of serum ionized calcium (Fig. 6).

In particular the increase in PTH release raises the serum calcium concentration toward normal ranges in three ways:

- increased bone resorption, which occurs within minutes after PTH secretion increases
- increased intestinal calcium absorption mediated by increased production of calcitriol, the most active form of vitamin D, which occurs at least a day after PTH secretion increases
- decreased urinary calcium excretion due to stimulation of calcium reabsorption in the distal tubule, which occurs within minutes after PTH secretion increases.

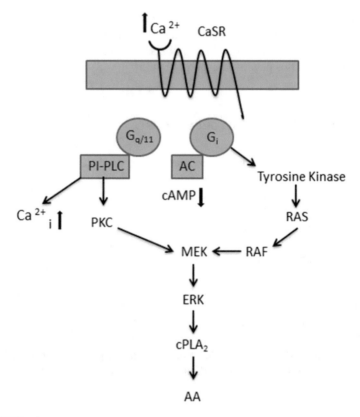

Fig. 6 PTH actions

On a more chronic basis, PTH also stimulates the conversion of calcidiol (25-hydroxyvitamin D) to calcitriol in renal tubular cells, thereby stimulating intestinal calcium absorption as well as bone turnover. Calcitriol inhibits PTH secretion through an indirect negative feedback which consists in its positive action on calcium levels; it also has a direct inhibitory action on PTH biosynthesis and parathyroid cell proliferation.

Skeletal Actions of PTH

PTH acts on bone, the main reservoir of calcium, to release calcium in two different phases [36]. The immediate effect of PTH is to mobilize calcium from skeletal stores that are readily available and in equilibrium with the extracellular fluid. Secondly PTH stimulates the release of calcium and phosphate by activation of bone resorption.

It is known that osteoblasts and not osteoclasts express PTH receptors, so osteoblasts are the main target for bone remodeling. However osteoclasts are indirectly activated in this process.

In fact, under PTH stimulation, pre-osteoblasts mature into bone-forming osteoblasts that produce collagen and subsequently mineralize matrix [37]. Since the remodeling unit is always coupled, once pre-osteoblasts are stimulated, they release cytokines that can activate osteoclasts resulting in bone resorption.

Thus, osteoclast formation requires an interaction with osteoblasts, which may depend upon cell to cell contact or regulators of osteoclast formation such as RANK (the receptor activator of nuclear factor kappa-B), osteoprotegerin, and RANK ligand (RANKL) [38]. PTH, then, can increase osteoclasts in number and activity indirectly through its effects on RANKL and osteoprotegerin [39].

New evidences suggest that PTH can actually bind osteoclasts through a different and incompletely characterized PTH receptor with specificity for the carboxyl-terminal region of PTH (C-PTHRs).

The net effect of PTH on bone can vary according to the severity and chronicity of the PTH excess. Chronic exposure to high serum PTH concentrations, typical of primary or secondary hyperparathyroidism, results in net bone reabsorption, whereas intermittent administration of recombinant human PTH (both full-length 1–84 or a 1–34 amino acids fragment) has been seen to stimulate bone formation more than resorption.

Moreover, specific elements of the PTH molecule seem essential for bone anabolism. PTH fragments 1–31 and 1–34 retain all of the biologic activity of the intact peptide; while amino-terminal truncation of the first two amino acids of PTH eliminates most of the cyclic adenosine monophosphate (cAMP) signaling, a pathway that seems important for the anabolic effect of PTH on bone [40, 41].

Secondary Hyperparathyroidism in ESRD

Secondary hyperparathyroidism (SHPT) is an adaptive and in many cases ultimately maladaptive process that develops in response to declining kidney function, impaired phosphate excretion, and failure to bioactivate vitamin D. Dysregulation of calcium and phosphorous homeostasis leads to decreased renal phosphate excretion, increased serum phosphorous, elevated levels of the phosphatonin fibroblast growth factor 23 (FGF-23), and reduced synthesis of calcitriol, the active form of vitamin D. These changes result into increased synthesis and secretion of parathyroid hormone (PTH) and parathyroid hyperplasia, contributing to the development of a vicious cycle.

Pathogenesis of SHPT

Continuous stimulation of the parathyroid glands because of a combination of elevated extracellular phosphate concentration, decreased extracellular ionized calcium concentration, and markedly reduced serum calcitriol leads to increased PTH synthesis and release. At the same time, elevated FGF-23 expression downregulates residual renal 25(OH)-1-hydroxylase, which exacerbates the effective deficiency of calcitriol, acting as an additional driver to SHPT. Even at early stages in the development of hyperparathyroidism, these changes are compounded of variable underexpression of the calcium-sensing receptor (CaSR) and vitamin D receptor (VDR), rendering the parathyroid cells unable to respond appropriately to ambient calcium and/or calcitriol. The resulting increase in proliferative activity in the parathyroid glands, eventually, leads to parathyroid hyperplasia.

Recent understanding of the molecular mechanisms behind phosphorous homeostasis has shown FGF-23 and its receptor fibroblast growth factor receptor 1 (FGFR1) to be important players [42]. Increases in both serum FGF-23 and PTH, in patients with chronic kidney disease (CKD), decrease the proximal tubular reabsorption of phosphate and maintain normo-phosphatemia in most patients until the GFR falls below 20 ml/min. Inevitably, as CKD progresses, these negative feedback loops are progressively sabotaged and eventually unable to maintain phosphate homeostasis.

Molecular Biology of Parathyroid Glands (Monoclonality)

As already mentioned in the previous chapters, PTH is synthesized as a precursor, the pre-pro-PTH, from which pro-PTH and the secreted form of PTH are then produced by two proteolytic cleavages. The pre-peptide is made of a central hydrophobic core and, often, charged amino acids at the N-terminal and C-terminal ends. The removal of the pre-peptide to produce pro-PTH is mediated by an enzyme associated with microsomes. After the cleavage the pre-peptide is rapidly degraded so that no labeled pre-peptide can be detected in biosynthetic cells. The proteolytic removal of the pre-peptide probably occurs before completion of the pro-PTH nascent chain, since pre-pro-PTH is difficult to detect in intact cells.

A comparison of the amino acid sequences of PTH showed a highly conserved PTH sequence among different species. In particular there are three regions relatively conserved: the first two regions enclose the biologically active site, in which an addition or loss of a single amino acid greatly reduces biological activity. This region is involved in binding of PTH to the receptor. The third region is located at the C-terminal side and it may have a biological effect on osteoclasts.

The PTH gene contains two introns that divide the gene into 3 exons that code, respectively, for a 5′ untranslated region (the signal peptide), PTH plus a 3′ untranslated region.

PTH, secreted as an 84 amino acid polypeptide, and a related molecule, parathyroid hormone-related protein (PTHrP), act on cells via a common G protein-coupled, seven-transmembrane helix receptor. The activated PTH1 receptor stimulates adenylyl cyclase and phospholipase C pathways.

The natural occurring PTH (1–37) fragment as well as PTH (1–34) maintains all the activities of the intact 1–84 hormone, since it has all the elements necessary to bind and activate PTH1 receptor. In particular the N-terminal region of the peptide is critical for full activation of the receptor; the N-terminal truncated peptide PTH (3–34) is a partial agonist while the further shortened peptide PTH (7–34) is a low affinity antagonist. Also, residues 17 to 31, near the C-terminal side of the PTH (1–34) are necessary for high affinity receptor binding.

PTHrP, physiologically produced in several tissues, is identical in sequence to PTH in the first 13 amino acids so it binds the same G-protein-coupled receptor and its N-terminal fragment has many functions that mimic those of full length PTHrP, PTH (1–34) and PTH (1–84).

In addition to the PTH1 receptor, another receptor named PTH2 has been identified. Its natural ligand, tuberoinfundibular peptide 39 (TIP39), is a structural PTH homolog. The PTH2 receptor shares 70% sequence similarity with the PTH1 receptor, but PTH1 receptor cannot be activated by TIP39 and PTH2 receptor does not respond properly to PTHrP. TIP39 binds to the PTH1 receptor, but its N-terminal domain is unable to stimulate cAMP accumulation, so it works as an antagonist at the PTH1 receptor.

The structure of human PTH (1–34) is a slightly bent helix while the PTH-PTHr complex structure is not fully determined yet.

PTH secretion is regulated by the extracellular calcium concentration, acting on calcium-sensing receptor (CaSR), a G-protein-coupled transmembrane receptor, mainly expressed on parathyroid chief cells, renal distal tubules and thyroid C-cells. CaSR signaling involves phospholipase C (PI-PLC), adenylate cyclase and mitogen-activated protein kinases (MAPK) pathways (ERK 1–2). When extracellular calcium concentration impairs, an acute secretory PTH response starts within few seconds and it can last for 60–90 min, increasing Ca^{2+} renal tubular reabsorption, Ca^{2+} releasing from bone and promoting 1,25(OH)2D3 synthesis in the renal proximal tubules, with increase in intestinal Ca^{2+} absorption.

CaSR, encoded by CaSR gene on chromosome 3 (3q13.3-21), has four main structural domains: a large NH2-terminal extracellular domain, a cysteine-rich domain linking the ECD to the first transmembrane helix, seven transmembrane domains and an intracellular COOH-terminal tail [43]. After its synthesis as a monomer, in the endoplasmic reticulum CaSR dimerizes through intermolecular disulfide bonds between cysteines 129 and 131 within each monomer; non-covalent hydrophobic interactions also contribute to the dimeric CaSR. Before reaching the cell surface, the receptor is glycosylated in the Golgi apparatus. This glycosylation seems to be necessary for right cell surface expression. The extracellular domain has a bilobed structure with a slot between the two lobes that contains the binding site for Ca^{2+}, called venus flytrap (VFT)-like motif. In absence of agonist, the VFT is open and it closes upon binding Ca^{2+}, with conformational changes in the TMD and intracellular domains that initiate signal transduction. When Ca^{2+} binds to CaSR, G proteins Gq/11, Gi, and G12/13 are activated and stimulate phospholipase C (PLC), inhibit adenylate cyclase, and activate Rho kinase, respectively (Fig. 7). CaSR can also lower cAMP indirectly by increasing intracellular Ca^{2+}, thereby reducing the activity of Ca^{2+}-inhibitable adenylate cyclase or activating phosphodiesterase [44]. Other intracellular signaling systems are involved in CaSR signaling, as ERK 1/2, phospholipases A2 and D, and the epidermal growth factor (EGF) receptor.

PTH secretion is regulated by calcium and phosphate, that regulate the gene expression and parathyroid proliferation too. Ca^{2+} and Pi PTH-regulation acts on PTH mRNA stability, with a post-transcriptional mechanism, by binding the protective trans acting parathyroid cytosolic proteins to a cis instability region in the 3′UTR. When serum Ca^{2+} concentration decreases, increased binding protects PTH mRNA from degradation by cytosolic ribonucleases, improving PTH secretion. When serum Pi concentration decreases, decreased binding stimulates an increased PTH mRNA degradation, impairing PTH secretion and its phosphaturic action. PTH mRNA binding proteins were purified by PTH RNA 3′-UTR affinity chromatography. One of these is identical to AU-rich binding factor (AUF1), involved in the stability of other mRNAs encoding for cytokines, oncoproteins and G-protein coupled receptors. The AUF1 stabilization mechanism is not clear

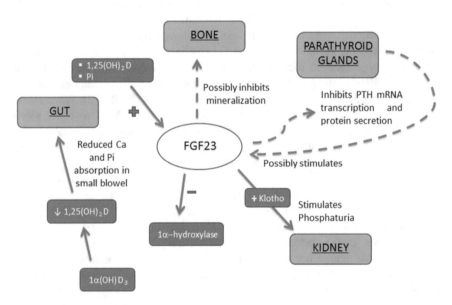

Fig. 7 Model for mechanisms for Ca^2-sensing receptor (CaR)-induced activation in the parathyroid cell. Activation of the 7-membrane-spanning CaR by extracellular Ca^{2+} results in Gq/11-mediated activation of phosphtidylinositol-phosphlipase C (PI-PLC), leading to intracellular Ca^2 ($Ca^{2+}i$) mobilization, protein kinase C (PKC) activation, and resultant stimulation of the mitogen-activating protein kinase (MAPK) cascade. The CaR also activates MAPK via an isoform of Gi protein, and subsequent downstream activation of a tyrosine kinase-dependent process, involving a RAS- and RAF-dependent series of steps. Activated MAPK then phosphorylates and activates $cPLA_2$, which releases free arachidonic acid (AA) that can be metabolized to biologically active mediators. MEK, ERK/MAPK kinase. AC, adenylate cyclase

(maybe post-translational). Other PTH mRNA binding proteins are hnRNP K. and Up stream of nras (UNR). Another protein, called dynein light chain or LC8 may play a role in the PTH mRNA intracellular localization in the parathyroid cells rather than in PTH mRNA stability.

PTH secretion is also regulated by 1,25-dihydroxyvitamin D [1,25(OH)2D3], that binds a specific PTH gene promoter sequence, called vitamin D response element (VDRE), reducing PTH gene transcription. VDR-RXR heterodimer binds to the VDRE, amplifying PTH-mRNA decrease. 1,25(OH)2D3 decreases PTH secretion also by increasing parathyroid VDR and CaSR concentrations. Calreticulin, a calcium binding protein, protects VDR-RXR from binding to VDRE.

Normally, parathyroid gland is in low turnover. Uremia, hypocalcemia, hyperphosphatemia and calcitriol deficiency induce parathyroid cells to divide by increasing cyclin/Cdk (cyclin dependent kinases) complexes and decreasing Cdk-inhibitors, that regulate mitotic division. Parathyroid hyperplasia is due to changes in the content of cell cycle regulators, like a cyclin D1 overexpression (also connected to human parathyroid adenomas).

In secondary hyperparathyroidism, initially glands growth is polyclonal and diffuse, then it may become monoclonal, with aggressive proliferation, maybe due to cyclin D1 overexpression. Monoclonal proliferation and tumorigenesis are also connected to many genetic factors, like protooncogene amplification (PRAD1/cyclin D1) and tumor suppressor reduction (p27Kip1).

Uremia-induced parathyroid mitoses are also connected and enhanced by high dietary P, meanwhile P restriction prevents parathyroid cells replication, counteracting uremia induced proliferative signals, but not inducing apoptosis. In uremia, parathyroid glands enlarge because of tissue hyperplasia rather than hypertrophy.

Studies in rats demonstrate that P-restriction increases serum calcitriol, that directly activates tumor suppressor p21 gene transcription, explicating an antiproliferative action. Other not known factors may produce post-transcriptional enhancement of p21 protein expression, contributing to its antiproliferative action. p21, with p27 and p57, explicates its function inhibiting G1-cyclin/cdk complexes and arresting G1 cell growth and binding to PCNA (proliferating nuclear cell antigen—a mitotic activity marker) trimers causing DNase-polymerase to lose processivity.

High-dietary P has not effects on p21 reduction; some other factors are involved in high-dietary P-induced parathyroid hyperplasia in uremia, such as TGFα, that increases in hyperplastic glands more in case of high dietary P rather than in case of low dietary P. TGFα induces cell growth through autocrine and paracrine mechanisms upon EGFR activation by the mature, soluble TGFα isoform, and through a juxtacrine pathway involving transmembrane TGFα isoform from an adjacent parathyroid cell. When activated, EGFR signaling involves a ras/MAPK activation that induces cyclin D1 and the cell cycle passes from G1 to S phase. Nuclear EGFR also works as a transcription factor, binding to adenosine-thymidine-rich regions in the cyclin D1 promoter, maybe explaining its high proliferating activity. In rat parathyroid glands, high dietary P enhances para-thyroid EGFR content, while low dietary P reduces EGFR levels.

Calcitriol explicates an antiproliferative action on parathyroid glands via VDR, inducing p21 and decreasing c-myc expression (that normally regulates the pro-gression from G1 to S phase in cell cycle); it limits the increase in parathyroid TGFα and EGFR, too. Therefore, in uremia, like the high dietary P, calcitriol deficiency and the development of a resistance to vitamin D action expose to an increased risk of parathyroid hyperplasia.

Monoclonality plays an important role in parathyroid tumorigenesis. Primary parathyroid hyperplasia, uremic parathyroid hyperplasia, MEN1-associated para-thyroid tumors and parathyroid carcinoma (rare) contain a monoclonal component. They all originate from a single clone that undergoes a genetic somatic mutation that leads to a proliferative advantage; then proliferating, other somatic mutations promote and sustain this uncontrolled proliferation. Parathyroid tumorigenesis involves many different factors, such as oncogenes, tumor suppressor genes and other mechanisms.

Among the involved oncogenes can be found PRAD1 (parathyroid adenomato-sis gene 1), cyclin D1, normally localized on long arm of chromosome 11 (11q13). In a small percentage of parathyroid tumors (5%), a pericentromeric inversion of an allele of chromosome 11 has been demonstrated, which results in a juxtapo-sition of the PRAD1 gene to the 5′ region of the PTH gene (11p15). As a con-sequence, the PRAD1 protein is overexpressed by stimulation by the PTH gene enhancers. Other oncogenes may be FGF-3, EGFR, KGFR (keratinocyte growth factor receptor) and RET proto-oncogene, whose germline missense mutation is involved in the MEN2A syndrome genesis (familial clustering of medullary thy-roid carcinoma, pheochromocytoma and parathyroid tumors), but not in sporadic parathyroid tumors [45].

When a bi-allelic inactivation of a tumor suppressor gene occurs, a proliferative advantage is triggered, by which cell proliferates in an uncontrolled manner. In most cases there is an inactivating point mutation of an allele, while other suffers a gross somatic deletion. This somatic deletion is heralded by allelic loss (LOH—loss of heterozygosity). In parathyroid tumors there are nonrandom, chromo-somal regions that display LOH and probably they host tumor suppressor genes. One of these regions is 13q11, MEN1 locus, involved in MEN1 syndrome and in sporadic benign parathyroid tumors. Inactivating mutations in the MEN1 gene result in loss of the gene product, menin, an inhibitor of the cyclin D1 prolifera-tive signal; a reduction of the menin in parathyroid tissue involves the binding of NF-kβ to the Cyclin D1 promoter, with an increase in its pro-proliferative activity. Another region showing LOH, in sporadic parathyroid tumors is 1p36, involved in MEN2A. Other tumor suppressor genes marginally involved in parathyroid tumor-igenesis could be p53, Rb.

Other molecular pathway could be also involved in parathyroid tumorigenesis, like microsatellite instability and telomerase activity.

References

1. Bliss RD, Gauger PG, Delbridge LW. Surgeon's approach to the thyroid gland: surgical anatomy and the importance of technique. World J Surg. 2000;24:891.
2. Akerström G, Malmaeus J, Bergström R. Surgical anatomy of human parathyroid glands. Surgery. 1984;95:14.
3. Wang C. The anatomic basis of parathyroid surgery. Ann 6. Surg. 1976;183:271.
4. Cernea CR, Brandão LG, Hojaij FC, De Carlucci D, Montentgro FL, Ploppper C. How to minimize complications in thyroid surgery? Auris Nasus Larynx. 2009;37(1):1–5.
5. Bliss RD, Gauger PG, Delbridge LW. Surgeon's approach to the thyroid gland: surgical anatomy and the importance of technique. World J Surg. 2000;24(8):291–7.
6. Gilmour JR. The gross anatomy of the parathyroid glands. J Pathol. 1938;46:133–49.
7. Akerstrom G, MalmaeusJ, Bergstrom R. Surgical anatomy of human parathyroid glands. Surgery. 1984;95:14–21.
8. Hojaij F, Vanderlei F, Plopper C, Rodrigues CJ, Jacomo A, Cernea C, Oliveira L, Marchi L, Brandao L. Parathyroid gland anatomical distribution and relation to anthropometric and demographic parameters: a cadaveric study. Anat Sci Int. 2011;86(4):204–12.
9. Som PM, Curtin HD. Head and Neck Imaging. 4th ed. St Louis, MO: Mosby; 2003.
10. Shen W, Düren M, Morita E, et al. Reoperation for persistent or recurrent primary hyperparathyroidism. Arch Surg. 1996;131:861.
11. Curley IR, Wheeler MH, Thompson NW, Grant CS. The challenge of the middle mediastinal parathyroid. World J Surg. 1988;12:818–24.
12. Norris EH. The parathyroid glands and the lateral thyroid in man: their morphogenesis, topographic anatomy and prenatal growth. Contrib Embryol. 1937;26:249–94.
13. Grant CS, van Heerden JA, Charboneau JW, James EM, Reading CC. Clinical management of persistent and/or recurrent primary hyperparathyroidism. World J Surg. 1986;10:555–65.
14. Salti GI, Fedorak I, Yashiro T, et al. Continuing evolution in the operative management of primary hyperparathyroidism. Arch Surg. 1992;127:831–7.
15. Udekwu AO, Kaplan EL, Wu T, Arganini M. Ectopic parathyroid adenoma of the lateral triangle of the neck: report of two cases. Surgery. 1987;101:114–8.
16. Thompson NW, Eckhanser FE, Harness JK. The anatomy of primary hyperparathyroidism. Surgery. 1982;92:814–21.
17. Cheung PSY, Borgstrom A, Thompson NW. Strategy in re operative surgery for hyperparathyroidism. Arch Surg. 1989;124:676–80.
18. Wheeler MH, Williams ED, WadeJSH. The hyperfunctioning intrathyroidal parathyroid gland: a potential pitfall in parathyroid surgery. World J Surg. 1987;11:110–14.
19. Billingsley KG, Fraker DL, Doppman JL, et al. Localization and operative management of undescended parathyroid adenomas in patients with persistent primary hyperparathyroidism. Surgery. 1994;116:982–90.
20. Carter WB, Carter DL, Cohn HE. Cause and current management of reoperative hyperparathyroidism. Am Surg. 1993;59:120.
21. Arveschoug AK, Brøchner-Mortensen J, Bertelsen H, Vammen B. Supernumerary parathyroid glands in recurrent secondary hyperparathyroidism. Clin Nucl Med. 2002;27:599.
22. Edis AJ, Levitt MD. Supernumerary parathyroid glands: implications for the surgical treatment of secondary hyperparathyroidism. World J Surg. 1987;11:398.
23. Mohebati A, Shaha AR. Anatomy of thyroid and parathyroid glands and neurovascular relations. Clin Anat. 2012;25(1):19–31.

24. Flament JB, Delattre JF, Pluot M. Arterial blood supply to the parathyroid glands: Implications for thyroid surgery. Surg Radiol Anat. 1982;3:279.
25. Drüeke T. The pathogenesis of parathyroid gland hyperplasia in chronic renal failure. Kidney Int. 1995;48:259–72.
26. Parfitt AM: The hyperparathyroidism of chronic renal failure: A disorder of growth. Kidney Int. 1997;52:3–9.
27. Silver J, Sela SB, Naveh-Many T. Regulation of parathyroid cell proliferation. Curr Opin Nephrol Hypertens. 1997;6:321–26.
28. Szabo A, Merke J, Beier E, Mall G, Ritz E. 1,25(OH)2 Vitamin D3 inhibits parathyroid cell proliferation in experimental uremia. Kidney Int. 1989;35:1045–56.
29. Tominaga Y, Tanaka Y, Sato K, et al. Histopathology, pathophysiology, and indications for surgical treatment of renal hyperparathyroidism. Semin Surg Oncol. 1997;13:78.
30. Matsuoka S, Tominaga Y, Sato T, et al. Relationship between the dimension of parathyroid glands estimated by ultrasonography and the hyperplastic pattern in patients with renal hyperparathyroidism. Ther Apher Dial. 2008;12:391.
31. Ritter H, Milas M. Parathyroidectomy: bilateral neck exploration. In: Terris D, editor. Operative techniques in Otolaryngology, St. Louis: Elsevier; 2009. p. 44.
32. Pattou FN, Pellissier LC, Noël C, et al. Supernumerary parathyroid glands: frequency and surgical significance in treatment of renal hyperparathyroidism. World J Surg. 2000;24:1330.
33. Nichol PF, Starling JR, Mack E, et al. Long-term follow-up of patients with tertiary hyperparathyroidism treated by resection of a single or double adenoma. Ann Surg. 2002;235:673.
34. Tominaga Y, Sato K, Tanaka Y et al. Histopathology and pathophysiology of secondary hyperparathyroidism due to chronic renal failure. Clin Nephrol. 1995;44(Suppl. 1):S42–47.
35. Martin LNC, Kayath MJ, Vieira JGH, Nose-Alberti V. Parathyroid glands in uraemic patients with refractory hyperparathyroidism: histopathology and p53 protein expression analysis. Histopathology. 1998;33:46–51.
36. Talmage RV, Mobley HT. Calcium homeostasis: reassessment of the actions of parathyroid hormone. Gen Comp Endocrinol. 2008;156:1.
37. Black DM, Greenspan SL, Ensrud KE, et al. The effects of parathyroid hormone and alendronate alone or in combination in postmenopausal osteoporosis. N Engl J Med. 2003;349:1207.
38. Yasuda H, Shima N, Nakagawa N, et al. Osteoclast differentiation factor is a ligand for osteoprotegerin/osteoclastogenesis-inhibitory factor and is identical to TRANCE/RANKL. Proc Natl Acad Sci U S A. 1998;95:3597.
39. Lee SK, Lorenzo JA. Parathyroid hormone stimulates TRANCE and inhibits osteoprotegerin messenger ribonucleic acid expression in murine bone marrow cultures: correlation with osteoclast-like cell formation. Endocrinology. 1999;140:3552.
40. Murrills RJ, Matteo JJ, Samuel RL, et al. In vitro and in vivo activities of C-terminally truncated PTH peptides reveal a disconnect between cAMP signaling and functional activity. Bone. 2004;35:1263.
41. Mohan S, Kutilek S, Zhang C, et al. Comparison of bone formation responses to parathyroid hormone (1-34), (1-31), and (2-34) in mice. Bone. 2000;27:471.
42. Galitzer H, Ben-Dov IZ, Silver J, Naveh-Many T. Parathyroid cell resistance to fibroblast growth factor 23 in secondary hyperparathyroidism of chronic kidney disease. Kidney Int. 2010;77:211–8.

43. Riccardi D, Brown EM. Physiology and pathophysiology of the calcium-sensing receptor in the kidney. Am J Physiol Renal Physiol. 2010;298:F485–99.
44. Zhang C, Miller CL, Brown EM, Yang JJ. The calcium sensing receptor: from calcium sensing to signaling. Sci China Life Sci. 2015;58(1):14–27.
45. Naveh-Many T. Molecular biology of the parathyroid. Kluwer Academic/Plenum publishers.

PTH Regulation by the Klotho/FGF23 Axis in CKD

Genta Kanai, Takatoshi Kakuta, Mario Cozzolino and Masafumi Fukagawa

The Parathyroid Gland

The parathyroid glands, first discovered by the Uppsala anatomist Ivear Sandstrom, appear as a pair of inferior and a pair of superior "bumps" on the dorsal side of the thyroid in adults [1]. The superior and inferior parathyroid glands are found in symmetrical positions in 80% and 70% of subjects, respectively. The parathyroid glands develop from the third and fourth pharyngeal pouches in humans between the fifth and twelfth weeks of gestation [2].

Normal adult parathyroid glands have a characteristic light yellow or red-brownish color and a soft consistency. Most glands are oval or bean-shaped, round, elongated, and bloated, and are multi lobulated. The normal gland size is 2–5 mm and weighs below 60 mg [3–5]. Autopsy studies revealed that 3–6% of normal individuals without hyperparathyroidism had fewer than four parathyroid glands and more than four glands were present in 2.5–6.7% of normal subjects, a condition called supernumerary glands. Supernumerary glands are defined as glands weighing more than 5 mg and located distant from the normal position and are usually found located in the thymus. Supernumerary glands occur in more than 10% of patients with multiple endocrine neoplasia (MEN) type 1 or secondary hyperparathyroidism (SHPT) [4–10].

G. Kanai · M. Fukagawa (✉)
Division of Nephrology, Endocrinology and Metabolism,
Tokai University School of Medicine, Tokyo, Japan
e-mail: fukagawa@tokai-u.jp

T. Kakuta
Division of Nephrology, Endocrinology and Metabolism,
Tokai University Hachioji Hospital, Hachioji, Japan

M. Cozzolino
Renal Division, ASST Santi Paolo e Carlo, Department of Health Sciences,
University of Milan, Milan, Italy

© Springer Nature Switzerland AG 2020
A. Covic et al. (eds.), *Parathyroid Glands in Chronic Kidney Disease*,
https://doi.org/10.1007/978-3-030-43769-5_2

21

The inferior thyroid artery primarily supplies the parathyroid glands, which is the primary vascular supply to both upper and lower parathyroid glands in 76–86% of subjects [11]. The parathyroid glands located low in the mediastinum may be supplied by a thymic branch of the internal mammary artery or by a branch of the aortic arch.

Physiology of the Parathyroid Glands

The main function of the parathyroid glands is to produce parathyroid hormone (PTH). PTH is one of three key hormones modulating calcium and phosphate homeostasis; being the other two calcitriol (1,25-dihydroxyvitamin D) and fibroblast growth factor 23 (FGF23) [12].

PTH is synthesized as a 115-amino acid polypeptide called pre-pro-PTH, which is cleaved within parathyroid cells at the amino-terminal portion, first to pro-PTH (90 amino acids) and then to PTH (84 amino acids). The 84-amino acids form is the stored, secreted and biologically active hormone. The biosynthetic process is estimated to take less than one hour while the secretion by exocytosis takes place within seconds after induction of hypocalcemia. Once secreted, PTH is rapidly cleared from plasma through uptake mainly by the liver and kidney: 1–84 PTH is cleaved into active amino- and inactive carboxyl-terminal fragments that are then cleared by the kidney. Intact PTH has a plasma half-life of two to four minutes while the carboxyl-terminal fragments have half-lives that are 5–10 times greater [13].

PTH Functions

The principal function of PTH is to maintain the extracellular fluid calcium concentration within a narrow normal range. The hormone acts directly on bone and kidney and indirectly on the intestine through its effects on synthesis of 1,25 OH2D to increase serum calcium concentration; in turn, PTH production is closely regulated by the concentration of serum ionized calcium (Fig. 1).

In particular the increase in PTH release raises serum calcium concentration toward normal ranges in three ways:

- increased bone resorption, which occurs within minutes after PTH secretion increases
- increased intestinal calcium absorption mediated by increased production of calcitriol, the most active form of vitamin D, which occurs at least a day after PTH secretion increases
- decreased urinary calcium excretion due to stimulation of calcium reabsorption in the distal tubule, which occurs within minutes after PTH secretion increases.

Fig. 1 PTH actions

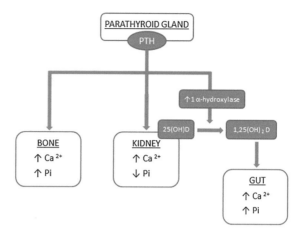

On a more chronic basis, PTH also stimulates the conversion of calcidiol (25-hydroxyvitamin D) to calcitriol in renal tubular cells, thereby stimulating intestinal calcium absorption as well as bone turnover. Calcitriol inhibits PTH secretion through an indirect negative feedback which consists in its positive action on calcium levels; it also has a direct inhibitory action on PTH biosynthesis and parathyroid cell proliferation [14].

Skeletal Actions of PTH

PTH acts on bone, the main reservoir of calcium, to release calcium in two different phases [15]. The immediate effect of PTH is to mobilize calcium from skeletal stores that are readily available and in equilibrium with the extracellular fluid. Secondly, PTH stimulates the release of calcium and phosphate by activation of bone resorption.

It is known that osteoblasts and not osteoclasts express PTH receptors, so osteoblasts are the main target for bone remodeling. However, osteoclasts are indirectly activated in this process [16]. In fact, under PTH stimulation, pre-osteoblasts mature into bone-forming osteoblasts that produce collagen and subsequently mineralize matrix [17]. Since the remodeling unit is always coupled, once pre-osteoblasts are stimulated, they release cytokines that can activate osteoclasts resulting in bone resorption.

Thus, osteoclast formation requires an interaction with osteoblasts, which may depend upon cell to cell contact or regulators of osteoclast formation such as RANK (the receptor activator of nuclear factor kappa-B), osteoprotegerin, and RANK ligand (RANKL) [18]. PTH, then, can increase osteoclasts in number and activity indirectly through its effects on RANKL and osteoprotegerin [19].

New evidences suggest that PTH can actually bind osteoclasts through a different and incompletely characterized PTH receptor with specificity for the carboxyl-terminal region of PTH (C-PTHRs) [16].

The net effect of PTH on bone can vary according to the severity and chronicity of the PTH excess. Chronic exposure to high serum PTH concentrations, typical of primary or secondary hyperparathyroidism, results in net bone reabsorption, whereas intermittent administration of recombinant human PTH (both full-length 1–84 or a 1–34 amino acids fragment) has been seen to stimulate bone formation more than resorption. Moreover, specific elements of the PTH molecule seem essential for bone anabolism. PTH fragments 1–31 and 1–34 retain all of the biologic activity of the intact peptide; while amino-terminal truncation of the first two amino acids of PTH eliminates most of the cyclic adenosine monophosphate (cAMP) signaling, a pathway that seems important for the anabolic effect of PTH on bone [20, 21].

Renal Actions of PTH

PTH stimulates calcium and phosphate reabsorption in the kidney and promotes the activation of calcidiol to calcitriol leading to an increase of intestinal calcium absorption and ultimately calcium blood levels.

Reabsorption of calcium—Filtered calcium is reabsorbed by a great part of the nephron. The mechanisms by which it is reabsorbed and their regulation, vary according to the function of location along the nephron. Most filtered calcium is reabsorbed passively in the proximal tubule due to the favorable electrochemical gradients created by sodium and water reabsorption. In contrast, calcium transport is actively regulated in the distal nephron according to the needs of the organism. This takes place in the cortical thick ascending limb of the loop of Henle (cTAL), as well as in the distal convoluted tubule (DCT) and adjacent connecting segment (a small segment between the distal tubule and cortical collecting tubule). PTH acts at both cTAL and DCT in the distal tubule to stimulate calcium reabsorption. Thus, if PTH secretion falls appropriately after an increase in serum ionized calcium, the ensuing fall in tubular calcium reabsorption and the increase in calcium excretion will contribute to restoring normocalcemia. High serum calcium itself also contributes to the calciuresis, acting via the CaSR [22, 23].

Reabsorption of phosphate—PTH, along with fibroblast growth factor 23 (FGF23), is a key hormonal determinant of serum phosphate concentration. It inhibits mostly proximal but also distal tubular reabsorption of phosphorus. This effect is primarily mediated by decreased activity, internalization and degradation of the Npt2A and Npt2C, sodium-phosphate cotransporters in the luminal membrane of the proximal tubules that mediate tubular reabsorption of phosphate.

Synthesis of calcitriol—PTH stimulates the synthesis of 1-alpha hydroxylase in the proximal tubules and, therefore, the conversion of calcidiol to calcitriol. Approximately 50 percent of patients with primary hyperparathyroidism show high serum calcitriol concentrations as a result of this action of PTH. PTH also decreases the activity of a 24-hydroxylase that inactivates calcitriol. This is an extremely important action of PTH in maintaining calcium homeostasis in states of vitamin D deficiency.

Other Actions of PTH

The possibility that PTH acts on other tissues has been raised in the attempt to explain certain clinical manifestations of primary and secondary hyperparathyroidism. Some experimental studies have found effects of PTH on the intestine, liver, adipose tissue, cardiovascular function, and neuromuscular function. Impaired glucose tolerance and alterations in lipid metabolism reminiscent of the metabolic syndrome have been described in hyperparathyroidism. Similarly, patients with primary hyperparathyroidism have an increased incidence of hypertension, left ventricular hypertrophy, and neuromuscular abnormalities. In addition, chronic excess of PTH, along with the associated elevations in the level of FGF23, has been implicated in the pathogenesis of vascular calcification and hypertension in patients with CKD [24, 25]. These atypical effects of PTH may be mediated by differing PTH moieties and/or differing PTH receptors [16]. Moreover, the extent to which these abnormalities improve after parathyroidectomy varies considerably, and whether they are actually directly caused by PTH excess is uncertain.

PTH Regulation and Pathophysiology of Secondary Hyperparathyroidism

PTH secretion is primarily regulated by extracellular calcium, along with extracellular phosphate, calcitriol, and fibroblast growth factor 23 (FGF23).

Extracellular calcium—The relationship between the serum calcium concentration and PTH secretion is described by an inverse, sigmoidal curve, based on studies of calcium-regulated PTH secretion both in vivo and in vitro [13, 26]. In normal individuals, a decrease in serum ionized calcium concentration of as little as 0.1 mg/dL (0.025 mmol/L) produces a large increase in serum PTH concentration within minutes; conversely, an equally small increase in serum ionized calcium rapidly lowers the serum PTH concentration. Particularly, PTH secretion steeply increases to a maximum value of five times the basal rate of secretion as calcium concentration falls from normal to the range of 1.9–2.0 mmol/L (7.5–8.0 mg/dl, measured as total calcium).

Parathyroid cells have many methods of adapting to increased needs for PTH production. The first most rapid (within minutes) being the secretion of preformed hormone in response to hypocalcemia. The second, within hours, are the changes in gene activity and increased PTH-mRNA are induced by sustained hypocalcemia. Finally, protracted challenge leads within days to cellular replication to increase glad mass.

The change in calcium concentration is perceived by an exquisitely sensitive calcium-sensing receptor (CaSR) on the surface of parathyroid cells.

When activated by a small increase in serum ionized calcium, the calcium-CaSR complex acts via one or more guanine nucleotide-binding (G) proteins through second messengers, to inhibit PTH secretion and decrease renal tubular reabsorption of calcium by the CaSR's actions on parathyroid and kidney, respectively. Conversely, the effect of deactivation of the receptor by a small decrease in serum ionized calcium concentration is to stimulate PTH secretion and enhance renal tubular reabsorption of calcium.

Calcium regulates not only the release but also the synthesis and degradation of PTH, in all its molecular forms. During hypocalcemia, intracellular degradation of PTH decreases, and a greater proportion of PTH 1–84 is secreted in relation with other molecular species of the hormone. In comparison, during hypercalcemia, intracellular degradation of intact PTH increases and reduces the availability of biologically active PTH 1–84 for secretion; consequently, mostly biologically inactive carboxyl-terminal fragments of PTH are secreted during hypercalcemia [12, 14, 27]. The ionized fraction of blood calcium is the most important determinant of hormone secretion. Magnesium may influence hormone secretion in the same direction as calcium. As a matter of fact, severe intracellular magnesium deficiency impairs PTH secretion. However, it is unlikely that physiologic variation in magnesium concentration affects PTH secretion.

Extracellular phosphate—Phosphate, like calcium, acts as an extracellular ionic messenger. Hyperphosphatemia, as well as extracellular calcium, calcitriol and FGF23, modulates many parameters of parathyroid function by stimulating PTH secretion, probably in large part by increasing PTH-mRNA stability and promoting parathyroid cell growth [28, 29]. These responses may be mediated, partially by the induction of hypocalcemia owing to the increase in serum phosphate concentration.

However, small elevations in serum phosphate concentrations may not be sufficient to lower serum calcium concentration to a level that stimulates PTH secretion. In addition, there is increasing evidence that hyperphosphatemia, regardless of calcium and calcitriol serum concentrations, directly stimulates PTH synthesis as well as parathyroid cellular proliferation in patients with advanced renal failure (the most common cause of hyperphosphatemia) [28, 29]. The nature of the putative phosphate-sensing mechanism is unknown, however, it has been recently demonstrated that phosphate can bind the CaR and interfere with the physiological inhibitory effect of calcium on PTH secretion (ref).

Calcitriol—Vitamin D is synthesized in the skin, or may be ingested in the diet, and is transported to the liver, where it is metabolized to form 25-hydroxyvitamin D (Fig. 2). 25-hydroxyvitamin D is the main storage form of vitamin D and is the substrate for the enzyme 1α-hydroxylase, which converts it into 1,25-dihydroxyvita-min D, the major circulating active metabolite of vitamin D. 1,25-dihydroxyvitamin D is responsible for the effects of vitamin D on calcium and phosphorus metabolism, the maintenance of bone health, and the regulation of the parathyroid glands [30, 31]. Parathyroid cells contain vitamin D receptors, and the PTH gene contains a vitamin D-response element. Calcitriol, by binding to the vitamin D receptor, inhibits PTH gene expression and, therefore, PTH synthesis [32]. Calcitriol also inhibits parathyroid cell proliferation. Some of the actions of calcitriol on parathyroid function are related to its ability to increase the expression of the CaSR.

FGF23—Fibroblast growth factor-23 (FGF23) is a 251-amino-acid protein (molecular weight: 26 kDa) that was found to be synthesized and secreted by osteocytes and osteoblasts [33]. FGF23 binds to and activates FGFR1, which is functional only if co-expressed with the Klotho transmembrane protein, as a Klotho-FGF receptor complex. When stimulated by phosphate increase and calcitriol elevation, FGF23 directly increases urinary fractional excretion of phosphate (FePi) in the proximal tubule by reducing the expression of type II sodium-phosphate cotransporters (NPT2a and NPT2c) and, indirectly it reduces phosphate absorption in the gut by suppressing 25-hydroxyvitamin D-1α-hydroxylase (1α-hydroxylase) activity.

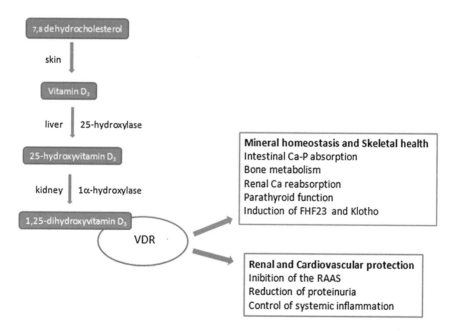

Fig. 2 Beneficial effects of VDR activation. Vitamin D actions require vitamin D activation to its hormonal form, 1,25-dihydroxyvitamin D, by renal and extrarenal 1a-hydroxylases to bind and activate the vitamin D receptor (VDR). Upon activation, ligand-bound VDR acts as a transcription factor to regulate the expression of genes involved in vitamin D maintenance of mineral homeostasis, skeletal health, renal and cardiovascular protection

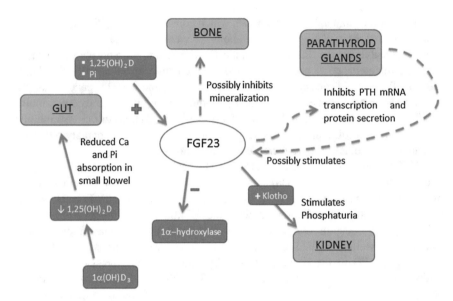

Fig. 3 FGF23 functions

In addition to its phosphaturic action, FGF23 exerts direct actions on parathyroid glands, inhibiting PTH synthesis and secretion [34] (Fig. 3). Therefore, PTH, calcitriol, and FGF23 all participate in maintaining both calcium and phosphate homeostasis.

Klotho

The Klotho gene encodes a single transmembrane protein belonging to glycosidase family 1 and is mainly expressed in the renal tubules [35, 36]. The Klotho protein forms a constitutive complex with several FGF receptor isoforms, such as FGFR1c, 3c, and 4 and markedly increases the specificity of FGFR for FGF23. That is, Klotho functions as a co-receptor for FGF23 [37]. The fact that FGF23 requires Klotho as a co-receptor is demonstrated by the finding that Klotho-deficient mice and FGF23-deficient mice have the same phenotype [38]. Extremely high serum FGF23 concentrations do not have adverse effects on Klotho-deficient mice, indicating that Klotho is required for FGF23 signaling [39].

Klotho is not a kidney-specific protein: Klotho mRNA is also expressed at high levels in the parathyroid gland, whereas it is barely expressed in the thyroid gland, intestinal tract, and liver. Immunohistochemical analyses have confirmed the specific localization of Klotho to the parathyroid gland and have also shown the presence of FGFR1 and FGFR3 in parathyroid tissue. These results provide further evidence that the parathyroid gland is the target organ of FGF23, due to the presence of FGFR-Klotho receptor complexes. Klotho is also expressed in other organs such as the brain, but it is particularly present in the distal convoluted tubules, in the proximal convoluted tubules and in the inner medullary collecting duct of the kidney [40]. In the kidney Klotho binds to the FGF receptor (FGFR) which in turn binds to FGF23 leading to the formation of a Klotho/FGFR/ FGF23 complex with subsequent activation of FGF23 signal trasduction. Klotho is required to convert different types of FGFR (FGFR1c, FGFR3c, FGFR4) into specific receptors for FGF23, increasing the affinity for it and not for other FGFs [41, 42].

There is also a soluble circulating form of Klotho which can still bind FGFRs but also functions as a humoral factor with pleiotropic activities including regulation of oxidative stress, growth factor signaling, and ion homeostasis [43]. Soluble Klotho can be generated in two ways: the extracellular domain of transmembrane Klotho can be shed by secretases and released into the circulation as cleaved Klotho; alternatively secreted Klotho can be generated by alternative transcript splicing. Interestingly soluble Klotho can bind to FGFR-FGF23 to form the active receptor complex but it seems to prevent high FGF23-induced effects [44]. In physiological conditions the kidney is the main responsible for the maintenance of Klotho homeostasis: it produces and releases cleaved Klotho and it also clears it from the blood through transcytosis in renal tubules. In patients with chronic kidney disease (CKD), as expected, Klotho levels are much lower than in healthy people and Klotho mRNA expression in the kidney decreases as GFR declines.

Klotho indirectly regulates PTH production through modulation of plasma levels of FGF23, active vitamin D and phosphate. In addition, membrane Klotho may have a direct effect on PTH production and release. Quantitative RT-PCR experiments have shown that Klotho mRNA is expressed at high levels in the parathyroid gland, whereas it is barely expressed in the thyroid gland, intestinal tract, and liver. Immunohistochemical analyses have confirmed the specific localization of Klotho to the parathyroid gland and have also shown the presence of FGFR1 and FGFR3 in parathyroid tissue. These results provide further evidence that the parathyroid gland is the target organ of FGF23, due to the presence of FGFR-Klotho receptor complexes. In physiological conditions FGF23 directly decreases PTH production and it also increases Klotho in the parathyroid gland, which facilitates its suppression of PTH production. Moreover, high vitamin D levels increase Klotho expression, which in turn promotes phosphaturia and suppresses 1,25 Vitamin D production [45].

Parathyroid Resistance to PTH and FGF23 Action in CKD

During CKD, the decrease in nephron number should activate the FGF23/αKlotho endocrine axis [46]. FGF23 is strictly involved in renal phosphate handling. When nephronic mass and GFR decrease, serum phosphate load on nephrons increases. Even in normo-phosphatemic CKD patients a positive phosphate balance occurs.

To counterbalance a phosphate overload, both FGF23 and PTH increase. Probably, CKD is the most common cause of chronically elevated serum FGF23 levels [47]; circulating FGF23 levels increase in parallel with the progressive fall in GFR and they can reach high and maladaptive concentrations in ESRD patients [48].

Klotho deficiency plays a major role in these responses. Klotho mRNA expression decreases progressively with GFR impairment, defining a reduction in serum klotho levels, starting from CKD stage 1. Serum Klotho reduction precedes serological elevation of FGF23, PTH and P. The progressive reduction of Klotho expression in renal and parathyroid tissue defines a FGF23 resistance state and an improvement in FGF23 synthesis [49].

Ben-Dov et al. reported Klotho expression in the parathyroid gland and showed that FGF23 significantly reduces *PTH* gene expression and PTH secretion by activating the mitogen-activated protein kinases (MAPK) pathway [50] or secondly through the Klotho-independent phospholipase C gamma (PLCγ)-dependent activation of the nuclear factor of activated T-cells (NFAT) cascade [51]. Experimental stimulation of activated FGF23 resulted in a rapid reduction in PTH expression and decreased PTH secretion. The decrease in serum PTH levels induced by FGF23 is partially reversed by MEK inhibition, indicating that the MAPK pathway is important for the suppression of PTH secretion by parathyroid FGF23-Klotho receptor complex signaling. FGF23 inhibits vitamin D metabolism, reduces serum phosphorus levels, and acts directly on the parathyroid gland to lower serum PTH levels. Thus, FGF23 targets the parathyroid gland and is involved in endocrine control signaling between bone cells and the parathyroid gland. Paradoxically, despite very high serum FGF23 levels in dialysis patients, PTH does not necessarily decrease [52, 53]. When FGF23 is administered to normal rats for 2 consecutive days, *PTH* mRNA significantly decreases in the parathyroid gland. However, in uremic rats with hyperparathyroidism, administration of FGF23 does not reduce *PTH* mRNA levels [27]. In vitro, the hyperplastic parathyroid gland secretes more PTH than the normal gland, but the addition of a significantly higher concentration of FGF23 does not reduce PTH secretion.

Galitzer et al. showed that rats with chronic kidney disease (CKD) are resistant to FGF23 in the parathyroid gland, indicating that CKD correlates with the downregulation of parathyroid Klotho and FGFR expression and FGF23 signaling [13]. *PTH* mRNA expression is known to be increased in CKD rats. Then, as CKD progresses into secondary hyperparathyroidism, Klotho and FGFR protein and mRNA levels decrease. In experiments investigating the response to FGF23 in the parathyroid gland of CKD rats, FGF23 administration did not decrease PTH expression in rats with advanced CKD at 6 weeks. Thus, Klotho and *FGFR* mRNA levels decrease in the parathyroid glands of CKD rats and Klotho and FGFR expression decrease in cultured glands in vitro. These results indicate that the increase in PTH expression in secondary hyperparathyroidism and the decrease in Klotho and FGFR expression are related to the resistance of the CKD rat parathyroid gland to FGF23.

Patients with secondary hyperparathyroidism maintain high serum PTH concentrations, but patients with uremia show extremely high FGF23 levels. To clarify the mechanism of resistance to FGF23 in uremic patients, Komaba et al.

investigated the expression of Klotho and FGFR in hyperplastic parathyroid tissue by immunohistochemistry [54]. Klotho and FGFR levels are significantly reduced in the hyperplastic parathyroid glands of uremic patients, when compared to normal tissues. These trends are more pronounced in tissues with advanced disease, accompanied by nodular hyperplasia.

These results answered some of the questions regarding the mechanism whereby serum PTH levels are resistant to extremely high serum FGF23 levels. Furthermore, it was shown that decreased levels of the Klotho-FGFR complex in the hyperplastic parathyroid gland may contribute to this resistance mechanism. This could explain the emergence of frameworks of SHPT. Despite its direct inhibitory action on the parathyroid, FGF23 also contributes to the progression of secondary hyperparathyroidism via reduction of renal calcitriol synthesis and subsequent decrease in active intestinal calcium and phosphate absorption [55].

References

1. Sandstrom IV. Omen ny kortel hos mennisken och atskilige baggdjur lakarefore rings (ed). Upsala. 1880;441–71.
2. Burke JF, Chen H, Gosain A. Parathyroid conditions in childhood. Semin Pediatr Surg. 2014;23:66–70.
3. Scharpf J, Randolph G. Thyroid and parathyroid glands, chapter 33. In: KJ Lee's, Chan Y, Goddard JC, editors. Essential otolaryngology. 11th ed. McGraw Hills Company Ltd. 2015.
4. Akerstrom G, Malmaeus J, Bergstrome R. Surgical anatomy of human parathyroid glands. Surgery. 1984;95:14–21.
5. Tominaga Y. Embryology and anatomy of parathyroid gland. In: Tominaga Y, editor. Surgery for hyperparathyroidism-forcusing on secondary hyperparathyroidism. Japan: TOKYO IGAKUSYA; 2017. p. 1–8.
6. Wang C. The anatomic basis of parathyroid surgery. Ann Surg. 1976;183:271–5.
7. Glmour JR. The gross anatomy of the parathyroid glands. J Pathol. 1938;46:1098.
8. Numano M, Tominaga Y, Uchida K, et al. Surgical significance of supernumerary parathyroid glands in renal hyperparathyroidism. Word J Surg. 2000;24:1330–4.
9. Pattou FN, Pellissier LC, Noel C, et al. Supernumerary parathyroid glands: frequency and surgical significance in treatment of renal hyperparathyroidism. World J Surg. 2000;24:1330–4.
10. Edis AJ, Purnell DC, van Heeden JA. The undecended "parathymus". An occasional cause of failed neck exploration for hyperparathyroidism. Ann Surg. 1979;190:64–8.
11. Alveryd A. Parathyroid glands in thyroid surgery. I. Anatomy of parathyroidglands. II. Postoperative hypoparathyroidism—Identification and autotransplantation of parathyroid glands. Acta Chir Scand. 1968;389:1–120.
12. Hasegawa H, Nagano N, Urakawa I, et al. Direct evidence for a causative role of FGF23 in the abnormal renal phosphate handling and vitamin D metabolism in rats with early-stage chronic kidney disease. Kidney Int. 2010;78:975–70.
13. Galitzer H, Ben-Dov IZ, Silver J, et al. Parathyroid cell resistance to fibroblast growth factor 23 in secondary hyperparathyroidism of chronic kidney disease. Kidney Int. 2010;77:211–8.
14. Portale AA, Booth BE, Halloran BP, et al. Effect of dietary phosphorus on circulating concentrations of 1,25-dihydroxyvitamin D and immunoreactive parathyroid hormone in children with moderate renal insufficiency. J Clin Invest. 1984;73:1580–9.

15. Almaden Y, Canalejo A, Hernandez A, et al. Direct effect of phosphorus on PTH secretion from whole rat parathyroid glands in vitro. J Bone Miner Res. 1996;11:970–6.

16. Moallem E, Kilav R, Silver J, et al. RNA-Protein binding and posttranscriptional regulation of parathyroid hormone gene expression by calcium and phosphate. J Biol Chem. 1998;273:5253–9.

17. Stubbs JR, Liu S, Tang W, et al. Role of hyperphosphatemia and 1,25-dihydroxyvitamin D in vascular calcification and mortality in fibroblastic growth factor 23 null mice. J Am Soc Nephrol. 2007;18:2116–24.

18. Silver J, Sela SB, Naveh-Many T. Regulation of parathyroid cell proliferation. Curr Opin Nephrol Hypertens. 1997;6:321–6.

19. Patel SR, Ke HQ, Vanholder R, Koenig RJ, Hsu CH. Inhibition of calcitriol receptor binding to vitamin D response elements by uremic toxins. J Clin Invest. 1995;96:50–9.

20. Patel S, Ke HQ, Vanholder R, Hsu CH. Inhibition of nuclear uptake of calcitriol receptor by uremic ultrafiltrate. Kidney Int. 1994;46:129–33.

21. Naveh-Many T, Rahamimov R, Livni N, Silver J. Parathyroid cell proliferation in normal and chronic renal failure rats. The effects of calcium, phosphate, and vitamin D. J Clin Invest. 1995;96:1786–93.

22. Mathias RS, Nguyen HT, Zhang MYH, Portale AA. Reduced expression of the renal calcium-sensing receptor in rats with experimental chronic renal insufficiency. J Amer Soc Nephrol. 1998;9(11):2067–74.

23. Kifor O, Moore FD, Wang P, Goldstein M, Vassilev P, Kifor I, et al. Reduced immunostaining for the extracellular Ca^{2+}-sensing receptor in primary and uremic secondary hyperparathyroidism. J Clin Endocrinol Metab. 1996;81:1598–606.

24. Roussanne MC, Lieberherr M, Souberbielle JC, Sarfati E, Drueke T, Bourdeau A. Human parathyroid cell proliferation in response to calcium, NPS R-467, calcitriol and phosphate. Eur J Clin Invest. 2001;31(7):610–6.

25. Chikatsu N, Fukumoto S, Takeuchi Y, Suzawa M, Obara T, Matsumoto T, et al. Cloning and characterization of two promoters for the human calcium-sensing receptor (CaSR) and changes of CaSR expression in parathyroid adenomas. J Biol Chem. 2000;275(11):7553–7.

26. Lundgren S, Carling T, Hjälm G, Juhlin C, Rastad J, Pihlgren U, et al. Tissue distribution of human gp330/megalin, a putative Ca^{2+}-sensing protein. J Histochem Cytochem. 1997;45:383–92.

27. Canalejo R, Canalejo A, MartinezMoreno JM, RodriguezOrtiz ME, Estepa JC, Mendoza FJ, et al. FGF23 fails to inhibit uremic parathyroid glands. J Amer Soc Nephrol. 2010;21(7):1125–35.

28. Densmore MJ, Sato T, Mannstadt M, et al. Interrelated role of Klotho and calcium-sensing receptor in parathyroid hormone synthesis and parathyroid hyperplasia. Proc Natl Acad Sci U S A. 2018.

29. Fukagawa M, Kaname S-Y, Igarashi T, Ogata E, Kurokawa K. Regulation of parathyroid hormone synthesis in chronic renal failure in rats. Kidney Int. 1991;39:874–81.

30. Dusso AS, Pavlopoulos T, Naumovich L, Lu Y, Finch J, Brown AJ, et al. P21 (WAF1) and transforming growth factor-alpha mediate dietary phosphate regulation of parathyroid cell growth. Kidney Int. 2001;59(3):855–65.

31. Cozzolino M, Lu Y, Finch J, Slatopolsky E, Dusso AS. P21 (WAF1) and TGF-alpha mediate parathyroid growth arrest by vitamin D and high calcium. Kidney Int. 2001;60(6):2109–17.

32. Gogusev J, Duchambon P, Stoermann-Chopard C, Giovannini M, Sarfati E, Drüeke TB. De novo expression of transforming growth factor-alpha in parathyroid gland tissue of patients with primary or secondary uraemic hyperparathyroidism. Nephrol Dial Transplant. 1996;11:2155–62.

33. Arcidiacono MV, Cozzolino M, Spiegel N, Tokumoto M, Yang J, Lu Y, et al. Activator protein 2alpha mediates parathyroid TGF-alpha self-induction in secondary hyperparathyroidism. J Am Soc Nephrol. 2008;19(10):1919–28.

34. Cordero JB, Cozzolino M, Lu Y, Vidal M, Slatopolsky E, Stahl PD, et al. 1,25-Dihydroxyvitamin D down-regulates cell membrane growth- and nuclear growth-promoting signals by the epidermal growth factor receptor. J Biol Chem. 2002;277(41):38965–71.

35. Mian IS. Sequence, structural, functional, and phylogenetic analyses of three glycosidase families. Blood Cells Mol Dis. 1998;24:83–100.

36. Kuro-o M, Matsumura Y, Aizawa H, Kawaguchi H, Suga T, Utsugi T, Ohyama Y, Kurabayashi M, Kaname T, Kume E, Iwasaki H, Iida A, Shiraki-Iida T, Nishikawa S, Nagai R, Nabeshima YI. Mutation of the mouse klotho gene leads to a syndrome resembling ageing. Nature. 1997;390(6655):45–51.

37. Kurosu H, Ogawa Y, Miyoshi M, Yamamoto M, Nandi A, Rosenblatt KP, Baum MG, Schiavi S, Hu MC, Moe OW, Kuro-o M. Regulation of fibroblast growth factor-23 signaling by klotho. J Biol Chem. 2006;281:6120–3.

38. Nakatani T, Sarraj B, Ohnishi M, Densmore MJ, Taguchi T, Goetz R, Mohammadi M, Lanske B, Razzaque MS. In vivo genetic evidence for klotho-dependent, fibroblast growth factor 23 (Fgf23)-mediated regulation of systemic phosphate homeostasis. FASEB J. 2009;23:433–41.

39. Urakawa I, Yamazaki Y, Shimada T, Iijima K, Hasegawa H, Okawa K, Fujita T, Fukumoto S, Yamashita T. Klotho converts canonical FGF receptor into a specific receptor for FGF23. Nature. 2006;444:770–4.

40. Sakaguchi K. Acidic fibroblast growth factor autocrine system as a mediator of calcium-regulated parathyroid cell growth. J Biol Chem. 1992;267:24554–62.

41. Matsushita H, Hara M, Endo Y, Shishiba Y, Hara S, Ubara Y, et al. Proliferation of parathyroid cells negatively correlates with expression of parathyroid hormone-related protein in secondary parathyroid hyperplasia. Kidney Int. 1999;55(1):130–8.

42. Lewin E, Garfia B, Almaden Y, Rodriguez M, Olgaard K. Autoregulation in the parathyroid glands by PTH/PTHrP receptor ligands in normal and uremic rats. Kidney Int. 2003;64(1):63–70.

43. Volovelsky O, Cohen G, Kenig A, Wasserman G, Dreazen A, Meyuhas O, et al. Phosphorylation of ribosomal protein S6 mediates mammalian target of rapamycin complex 1-induced parathyroid cell proliferation in secondary hyperparathyroidism. J Am Soc Nephrol. 2016;27(4):1091–101.

44. Gunther T, Chen ZF, Kim J, Priemel M, Rueger JM, Amling M, et al. Genetic ablation of parathyroid glands reveals another source of parathyroid hormone. Nature. 2000;406(6792):199–203.

45. Correa P, Akerstrom G, Westin G. Underexpression of Gcm2, a master regulatory gene of parathyroid gland development, in adenomas of primary hyperparathyroidism. Clin Endocrinol (Oxf). 2002;57(4):501–5.

46. Morito N, Yoh K, Usui T, Oishi H, Ojima M, Fujita A, et al. Transcription factor MafB may play an important role in secondary hyperparathyroidism. Kidney Int. 2018;93(1):54–68.

47. Naveh-Many T, Silver J. Transcription factors that determine parathyroid development power PTH expression. Kidney Int. 2018;93(1):7–9.

48. Arnold A, Brown MF, Ureña P, Gaz RD, Sarfati E, Drüeke TB. Monoclonality of parathyroid tumors in chronic renal failure and in primary parathyroid hyperplasia. J Clin Invest. 1995;95:2047–54.

49. Chudek J, Ritz E, Kovacs G. Genetic abnormalities in parathyroid nodules of uremic patients. Clin Cancer Res. 1998;4:211–4.

50. Ben-Dov IZ, Galitzer H, Lavi-Moshayoff V, Goetz R, Kuro-o M, Mohammadi M, Sirkis R, Naveh-Many T, Silver J. The parathyroid is a target organ for FGF23 in rats. J Clin Invest. 2007;117(12):4003–8.

51. Falchetti A, Bale AE, Amorosi A, Bordi C, Cicchi P, Bandini S, Marx SJ, Brandi ML. Progression of uremic hyperparathyroidism involves allelic loss on chromosome 11. J Clin Endocrinol Metab. 1993;76:139–44.

52. Gutierrez O, Isakova T, Rhee E, Shah A, Holmes J, Collerone G, Jüppner H, Wolf M. Fibroblast growth factor-23 mitigates hyperphosphatemia but accentuates calcitriol deficiency in chronic kidney disease. J Am Soc Nephrol. 2005;16:2205–15.
53. Larsson T, Nisbeth U, Ljunggren O, Jüppner H, Jonsson KB. Circulating concentration of FGF-23 increases as renal function declines in patients with chronic kidney disease, but does not change in response to variation in phosphate intake in healthy volunteers. Kidney Int. 2003;64:2272–9.
54. Komaba H, Goto S, Fujii H, et al. Depressed expression of Klotho and FGF receptor 1 in hyperplastic parathyroid glands from uremic patients. Kidney Int. 2010;77:232–8.
55. Tahara H, Imanishi Y, Yamada T, Tsujimoto Y, Tabata T, Inoue T, Inaba M, Morii H, Nishizawa Y. Rare somatic inactivation of the multiple endocrine neoplasia type 1 gene in secondary hyperparathyroidism of uremia. J Clin Endocrinol Metab. 2000;85:4113–7.

Parathyroid Imaging in Patients with Renal Hyperparathyroidism

Elif Hindié, Pablo A. Ureña-Torres and David Taïeb

Pathophysiology of Renal Hyperparathyroidism

Secondary hyperparathyroidism (sHPT) is a frequent and major complication in patients with end-stage renal disease on long-term haemodialysis or peritoneal dialysis [1]. With the decline of kidney function, sHPT develops due to a combination of factors, including hyperphosphatemia, elevated FGF-23 (Fibroblast Growth Factor-23) levels, reduced 1alpha-hydroxylation of vitamin D and the consequent tendency towards hypocalcemia. In patients on long-standing dialysis, the chronic parathyroid stimulation leads to parathyroid enlargement progressing from diffuse hyperplasia of the parathyroid glands to asymmetrical nodular and tumor-like monoclonal growth and eventually to functional autonomy due to the decrease in expression of vitamin D receptor and calcium sensing receptor on the parathyroid cells.

sHPT is associated with increased risk of cardiovascular events and death [2–6]. The arsenal of medical treatment includes dietary phosphorus restriction, phosphate binders, vitamin D sterols and analogs, and calcimimetics. The use of calcimimetics has increased the likelihood of achieving the targets set by either the National Kidney Foundation's Kidney Disease Outcomes Quality Initiative (NKF-K/DOQI™) [7], or the Kidney Disease Improving Global Outcomes

E. Hindié (✉)
Department of Nuclear Medicine, Haut-Lévêque Hospital, CNRS-UMR 5287, Translational and Advanced Imaging Laboratory (TRAIL), University of Bordeaux, Bordeaux, France
e-mail: elif.hindie@chu-bordeaux.fr

P.A. Ureña-Torres
AURA Nord Saint Ouen, Department of Dialysis and Department of Renal Physiology, Necker Hospital, University of Paris Descartes, Paris, France

D. Taïeb
Department of Nuclear Medicine, La Timone Hospital, CERIMED, Aix-Marseille University, Marseille, France

© Springer Nature Switzerland AG 2020
A. Covic et al. (eds.), *Parathyroid Glands in Chronic Kidney Disease*,
https://doi.org/10.1007/978-3-030-43769-5_3

(KDIGO^{TM}) [8], and has reduced the number of patients referred to PTx. However, in the "EVOLVE" trial, that included 3,883 hemodialysis patients, cinacalcet (Sensipar/Mimpara, Amgen) did not significantly reduce the risk of death [9].

Following renal transplantation, patients with parathyroid hyperplasia may develop transient hypercalcemia that gradually resolves with the decrease in PTH secretion and the involution of parathyroid hyperplasia. In more than 10% of patients, however, HPT persists and is named tertiary HPT (tHPT) [10, 11].

Surgery for Renal Hyperparathyroidism

When medical treatment of sHPT fails, or is associated with severe intolerance and undesirable side effects, parathyroidectomy (PTx) becomes necessary [12, 13]. Based on NKF/K-DOQI (National Kidney Foundation/Kidney-Disease Outcomes Quality Initiative) guidelines, patients with PTH levels >800 pg/ml, with hypercalcemia and/or hyperphosphatemia—or a raised calcium/phosphate (CaxP) product—despite medical therapy should be offered PTx [7]. Other strong indications for surgery are the presence of complications, such as intractable pruritus, bone pain, spontaneous tendon and bone fractures, metastatic calcifications, and calciphylaxis [14–17].

Surgery can also be needed in patients with persistent hyperparathyroidism after renal transplantation (tHPT) [18]. Treatment of tHPT is mandatory since persistently elevated PTH concentrations after kidney transplantation increase the risk of renal allograft dysfunction and osteoporosis. Several studies suggested that PTx is the treatment of choice for tHPT [10, 11].

Many studies, mostly observational, have shown that parathyroid surgery is associated with a beneficial impact on classical symptoms and signs of sHPT as well as on hard clinical outcomes such as fractures, bone mineral density, vascular calcification, cardiovascular mortality and morbidity [12, 18]. Parathyroidectomy has proved to be effective in reducing elevated levels of PTH, calcium, phosphorus, CaxP product, and FGF-23, for improving symptoms, bone mass, anemia, hypertension, cardiac hypertrophy, and for reducing mortality [14, 17, 19]. Quality of life is also improved [20].

The successful outcome of PTx (i.e. HPT suppression without hypoparathyroidism) is very dependent on the skills and experience of the surgeon. The surgeon will explore the four glands and either perform subtotal PTx (leaving a small part of one gland with its blood supply) or total PTx with auto-transplantation (AT) of small pieces of parathyroid tissue (grafts) in a muscle of the forearm or neck (PTx + AT). Most surgeons will also routinely perform a trans-cervical bilateral thymectomy. With this standard surgery, and in the absence of preoperative imaging, the rates of persistent HPT and that of permanent hypoparathyroidism (due to loss of blood supply to the remnant) are about 5–10% and 5–20%, respectively [21–23]. During long-term follow-up, disease recurrence may be observed in about 20–30% of patients [21, 23]. Total PTx without transplantation can somewhat lower the overall failure rate; it is, however, associated with higher rates of permanent hypoparathyroidism, and is therefore not favored by nephrologists due to the risk of adynamic bone disease [23].

Ectopic Glands and Supranumerary Parathyroids

The parathyroid glands develop from the 3rd and 4th pharyngeal pouches. The 3rd pouch differentiate into the thymus and inferior parathyroid glands (PIII), whereas the fourth pouches yield the superior parathyroid glands (PIV). Normal parathyroid glands are roughly the size of a lentil and their individual weight is 35–50 mg.

Parathyroid surgery of sHPT requires identification of all parathyroid glands and considering the possibility of ectopic or supernumerary glands.

The risk of ectopia of one or more parathyroid glands is not rare [24]. Although the majority of ectopic glands present a minor ectopia (e.g., in thyrothymic ligaments, tracheo-esophageal groove or partially embedded in the thyroid) and should be easily located by an experienced surgeon, some present major ectopia (e.g., low mediastinal, retro-esophageal, inside carotid sheath, submandibular/ undescended, strictly intrathyroidal), which might lead to surgery failure, even for experienced surgeons.

Supranumerary parathyroids can be present in 10–15% of individuals [25]. The continuous stimulation encountered in renal hyperparathyroidism can affect any supranumerary or even rudimentary parathyroid tissue and lead to a high rate of macroscopically detectable and clinically significant supranumerary glands. Supranumerary parathyroid glands can also be located in eutopic retrothyroid position but also often so in the thymus. They can also be ectopically located within the carotid sheath, alongside the vagus nerve, low in the mediastinum, or in intrathyroidal location.

Ultrasonography

Ultrasonography (US) is inexpensive, widely available and does not require exposure to ionizing radiation. High-resolution ultrasonography (US) with a probe of 7.5 or 10 MHz is often used in first-line parathyroid imaging. Normal parathyroid glands are usually invisible on US. Abnormal parathyroid glands appear as well-demarcated hypoechogenic ovoid nodules in contrast to the hyperechoic thyroid tissue. They are usually solid, but large parathyroids may have a cystic component. US also provides information on the thyroid gland and vasculature of adenomas. US can accurately define the size and structure of parathyroid glands as well as differentiate diffuse and nodular hyperplasia [26]. US may be also useful to predict the response of SHPT to vitamin D analogs and cinacalcet and to assess for regression of parathyroid glands hyperplasia by measurement of parathyroid gland volume [27]. However, the quality of US is largely dependent on the radiologist's experience and patient's body habitus. Moreover, small lesions and the majority of ectopic glands can be missed by US [28]. Posterior adenomas located in the tracheoesophageal groove as well as those located behind the clavicles or sternum can be masked by the acoustic shadow.

99mTc-sestamibi (MIBI) scintigraphy has higher sensitivity at detecting ectopic parathyroids compared to ultrasonography [29–34]. Moreover, recent hybrid gamma cameras now allow delineating the precise anatomical position of ectopic glands by fusing three-dimensional 99mTc-sestamibi images with CT cross-sectional images (SPECT/CT) [35].

Parathyroid Scintigraphy

SestaMIBI (methoxyisobutylisonitrile) radiolabeled with technetium-99m (^{99m}Tc-MIBI) is used in parathyroid scintigraphy protocols. The tracer is not specific for parathyroid tissue and is also taken up by thyroid tissue. However, differentiating parathyroid lesions from thyroid uptake is possible via one of two means: (1) delayed acquisition which demonstrates a prolonged retention within hyperfunctioning parathyroid glands (single tracer-dual-phase protocol); (2) subtraction of thyroid image by using an additional thyroid tracer (dual tracer-subtraction protocol).

In essence the single-tracer approach is based on differential ^{99m}Tc-MIBI retention between parathyroid and thyroid tissue [36, 37]. ^{99m}Tc-MIBI retention is prolonged in parathyroid lesions whereas the tracer washes out more rapidly from normal thyroid tissue. The original dual-phase protocol requires only two planar images, one recorded early (15 minutes) and the other late (2–3 hours) after ^{99m}Tc-MIBI injection [36, 38]. Focal areas showing an increase in uptake over time (relative to the thyroid) are suggestive of parathyroid lesions. However, parathyroid lesions with rapid tracer clearance can be missed. Several hypotheses have been raised to explain this rapid wash-out from some parathyroid lesions, such as overexpression of ^{99m}Tc-MIBI efflux proteins, fewer mitochondrial-rich oxyphil cells or low active growth phase.

The optimal "dual-tracer" protocol uses ^{99m}Tc-MIBI and iodine-123. The main advantage of using ^{123}I as a thyroid tracer is that thyroid and parathyroid images can be acquired simultaneously in a dual energy window set-up [39, 40]. ^{123}I is usually injected two hours before ^{99m}Tc-MIBI. The pinhole acquisition can start 3–5 min after ^{99m}Tc-MIBI injection. After acquisition, the ^{123}I thyroid image is digitally subtracted from the ^{99m}Tc-MIBI image. The residual foci correspond to the hyperfunctioning parathyroid glands (Fig. 1a). Technetium-99m pertechnetate (^{99m}TcO$_4$−) is less suitable as a thyroid tracer for parathyroid scintigraphy. Because it uses the same radionuclide as ^{99m}Tc-MIBI and simultaneous acquisition is not possible. The thyroid image is thus acquired either before or after

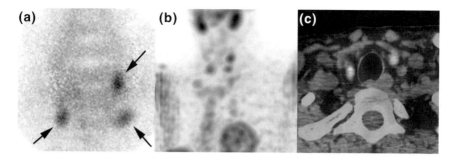

Fig. 1 Secondary HPT. 99mTc-sestaMIBI/123I subtraction parathyroid scintigraphy shows high uptake of 99mTc-sestaMIBI in 3 parathyroid glands (arrows) (**a** pinhole, **b** MIP image, **c** subtraction SPECT/CT centered over the inferior parathyroid glands). The results suggest that the right superior gland (barely visible) is the least active (autonomous) gland and can be selected for remnant or parathyroid tissue transplantation. This should insure preservation of parathyroid function while reducing the risk of recurrence

[99mTc-MIBI]99mTc-MIBI image acquisition. Patient motion between these two acquisitions may lead to artifacts on the subtraction images.

Although no comparative studies have been performed in sHPT, several recent prospective comparative studies have shown the superiority of dual-tracer subtraction imaging over dual-phase imaging in primary hyperparathyroidism, whether at initial operation or in re-operative cases, with a gain in at least 20% in sensitivity [41–46].

Pinhole view is necessary for optimal sensitivity [43, 44, 47]. Moreover, image subtraction needs to be used carefully and progressively in order to avoid clearance of smaller glands [47]. Dual-tracer imaging should be performed at least three weeks after radiologic examinations involving iodine contrast media administration. Also, thyroid hormone replacement therapy should be withheld for two weeks before imaging. This is necessary even in case of previous thyroidectomy as [123]123I would allow the correct identification of thyroid remnants. When possible, vitamin D derivatives and calcimimetics should be withdrawn before scintigraphy (for at least 1 week) in order to enhance tracer uptake and sensitivity.

Regardless of the protocol used, the examination needs to cover a large anatomical view, from the angle of the mandible to the upper part of the myocardium because ectopic adenomas may be widely distributed [47]. Therefore, either a large-field of view planar image or a cervico-mediastinal SPECT/CT should follow pinhole acquisition in order not to miss ectopic glands.

SPECT/CT is less sensitive than pinhole acquisition in the thyroid bed area, but it provides precise anatomical position of glands, and their size, and increases diagnostic confidence in doubtful situations. Images of [99mTc-MIBI]99mTc-MIBI and iodine-123 "dual-tracer" SPECT/CT can be displayed side by side. Subtraction can also be performed on SPECT/CT images (Fig. 1c).

Role of Preoperative Imaging in Renal Hyperparathyroidism

Whatever the surgical procedure that is performed (e.g., subtotal PTx or total PTx with autotransplantation), identification by the surgeon of all parathyroid tissue is required. This is sometimes difficult. In a recent study, 12.8% of patients had less than 4 parathyroid glands identified at surgery and, this was associated with the risk of persistent hyperparathyroidism [48]. This is also consistent with a large retrospective analysis showing that in about 10% of operated patients, PTH levels at 1 month remained highly elevated ($\geq$897 pg/mL) [49]. Difficulty at identifying all parathyroid glands is also associated with a higher risk of surgical complications, such as injury to the recurrent laryngeal nerve [50]. These factors are important to consider as parathyroid surgery in the setting of renal hyperparathyroidism is known to be associated with higher risk of morbidity than in the setting of primary hyperparathyroidism [51].

Because bilateral cervicotomy is required, the role of preoperative imaging studies prior to initial surgery for sHPT remains controversial [52]. However, preoperative imaging can be of help with the:

1. Identification of orthotopic enlarged parathyroid glands in the neck with distinction between thyroid nodules from nodular parathyroid hyperplasia.
2. Localization of ectopic and supernumerary parathyroid glands that are present in up to 25% of patients.
3. Choice of the most appropriate parathyroid gland for preservation.

Failure to identify four parathyroid glands usually results in persistent HPT [22, 48]. The identification of all parathyroid tissue depends on the experience of the surgeon. It is not unusual for parathyroid glands to show some asymmetrical positioning on both sides of the neck. Furthermore, some parathyroid glands can be small in size after calcimimetics. Extensive surgical dissection would increase operative time and also increase the risk of morbidity (hematoma, recurrent laryngeal nerve palsy, necrosis of the glandular remnant and hypoparathyroidism) [50]. This is particularly true in these patients who are at bleeding risk, and at risk of other complications [51]. When less that 4 glands are identified during the exploration, the information provided by preoperative scintigraphy may potentially modify the area of surgical exploration and reduce operating time and complications. Identifying all four parathyroid glands in patients with sHPT can also be difficult due to the high prevalence of nodular goiter in this patient population and the gross appearance of hyperplastic glands that may mimic thyroid tissue. Parathyroid scintigraphy, when performed as a dual tracer protocol may facilitate the distinction between thyroid and parathyroid nodular tissue.

Even in experienced hands, the inability to identify an ectopic or supernumerary parathyroid may occur and is the main cause of failure, persistence or early recurrence of sHPT [53]. The high rate of detection of ectopic parathyroid glands is probably the most important contribution that preoperative imaging can make.

Tha ability to detect ectopic parathyroid glands is considered the main advantage of PS over neck US [33]. SPECT/CT acquisition now allows delineating the precise anatomical position of ectopic glands [54]. A supernumerary "fifth" parathyroid gland is present in about 10–15% of individuals and some patients may have >5 hyperplastic glands. About half of these glands are located in the thymus. Some studies using dual-isotope ^{123}I/^{99m}Tc-SestaMIBI subtraction scintigraphy, or dual-phase imaging with additional pinhole or SPECT acquisition, identified macroscopic supernumerary parathyroid glands before initial surgery [33, 34, 55, 56]. The dual-phase protocol with only parallel-hole imaging rarely identifies all four parathyroid glands [57, 58] and it is thus difficult to state if one of the identified foci corresponds to a supernumerary gland.

Besides depicting ectopic and/or supernumerary gland, 99mTc-sestamibi scanning can offer functional information that can be helpful to select the remnant parathyroid tissue with the least autonomy, thus reducing the risk of recurrence [34, 59, 60]. Preservation of some parathyroid tissue is needed to maintain a correct mineral balance and avoid adynamic bone disease. The optimal volume to be preserved as a glandular remnant or grafted tissue should be slightly above that of a normal parathyroid gland (about 60 mg). The choice of the gland depends on its gross appearance (the gland should be less likely to have severe nodular hyperplasia) as well as its anatomical situation [15]. The functional information provided by parathyroid scintigraphy may guide surgeons towards the most suitable gland for preservation (least active/autonomous) [33, 34, 37, 59] (Fig. 1). In a retrospective analysis, a higher rate of recurrence was observed when remnant tissue was selected from a parathyroid gland with high ^{99m}Tc-SestaMIBI uptake [59]. The value of other tracers such as fluorocholine (FCH) PET/CT in this regard is largely unknown.

Overall, a randomized controlled study designed to assess the impact of PS on the rate of persistence, morbidity, and recurrence of sHPT would be of particular interest.

For tHPT, When the disease is limited to one or two glands, patients may benefit from more limited resection [61]. However, this should be the case only in carefully selected patients since this strategy can be associated with increased risk of persistent/recurrent disease [62].

Imaging Strategy Before Reoperation for Persistent or Recurrent Hyperparathyroidism

Persistent sHPT diagnosed in the early post-operative period, or during the first six months, usually results from missed orthotopic or ectopic glands, or supernumerary macroscopic parathyroid glands. Delayed recurrences due to growth of the remaining parathyroid tissue (from remnant/grafts) or supernumerary glands are sometimes observed after an appropriate initial PTx; this rate can reach 20–30%

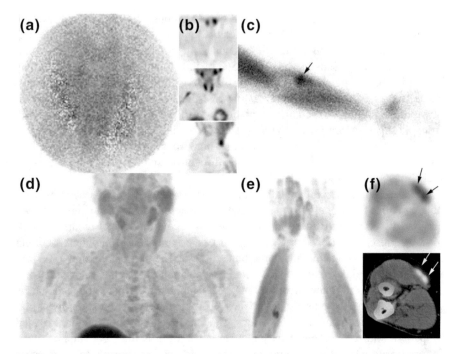

Fig. 2 Secondary HPT with recurrence due to hyperplasia of forearm grafts. 99mTc-sestaMIBI/123I subtraction parathyroid scintigraphy (**a** to **c**) and Fulorocholine PET/CT (**d** to **f**) showed abnormal uptake in the forearm (arrows) without any additional abnormality on cervico-mediastinal images (**a** planar pinhole subtraction, **b** SPECT, **d** FCH MIP image)

after 5 years of continuing dialysis [14, 21, 23]. Imaging before reoperation for recurrence should thus also assess the parathyroid remnant in the neck or the site of the autotransplant (Fig. 2).

Interestingly, patients who are referred for imaging of "recurrent HPT" not infrequently harbor two sites of autonomous disease [63]: one corresponding to a recurrence that developed within the preserved tissue and one corresponding to a supernumerary parathyroid (Fig. 3). Thus recurrent sHPT can be due to hyperplasia of the subtotally resected parathyroid gland or autograft in forearm, a supernumerary parathyroid gland, or both [63].

Recurrence may also rarely develop from parathyromatosis. Parathymosis in a previous surgical field, results from growth of parathyroid nests following accidental cell grafting (e.g., rupture of the parathyroid capsule of a cystic parathyroid, with spillage of parathyroid cells in the surgical field). In these situations, PS shows multiple hyperfunctioning foci [63].

Reoperative parathyroid surgery is challenging with higher risks of complications than initial surgery. A combination of imaging techniques (ultrasound, 99mTc-sestamibi/iodine-123 subtraction, CT, MRI, fluorocholine PET/CT) is sometimes necessary to localize the offending lesion with enough certainty. This is

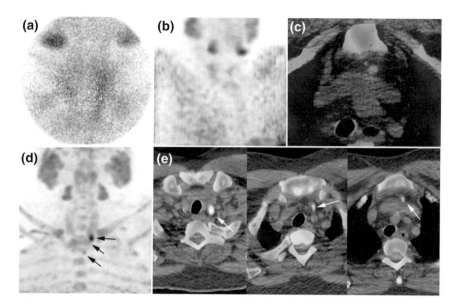

Fig. 3 Recurrent secondary HPT with multiple hyperplastic glands. Absence of significant foci on PS **a** planar pinhole, **b** MIP, **c** subtraction SPECT/CT showing a small nodule located in the anterosuperior mediastinum without significant uptake. FCH PET/CT revealed 3 nodules located in the lower neck and upper mediastinum (arrows) corresponding to a left hyperplasic PIII gland and 2 additional supranumerary parathyroid glands (**d** MIP, **e** PET/CT fusion images centered over the 3 nodules)

the case for reoperation in renal hyperparathyroidism as well as in reoperation for primary hyperparathyroidism. Figures 4 and 5 show examples of ectopic parathyroid glands with correlation between two imaging modalities (Figs. 4 and 5).

Parathyroid 4D-CT Scan

4D-CT is used mainly as a second line imaging modality in ectopic or re-operative surgery (Fig. 4). Because 4D-CT scanner uses a 3- or a 4-phase CT protocol, it delivers a high dose to the thyroid, which is problematic in younger patients [64], and needs the injection of contrast medium.

Parathyroid Imaging with Novel Pet Tracers

Besides 99mTc-sestamibi imaging, some radiopharmaceuticals labelled with positron emitters can be helpful for parathyroid imaging such as 11C-methionine, 11C-choline and 18F-fluorocholine (FCH) [54, 65–67].

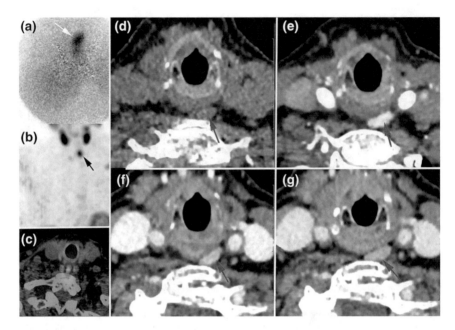

Fig. 4 Congenital ectopia of PIV. Concordance between PS (**a** subtraction pinhole, subtraction MIP, subtraction SPECT/CT) and 4D CT (**d** unenhanced, **e** arterial, **f** early venous phase image and **g** delayed venous phase image) for a left retrocricoid PIV adenoma (arrows)

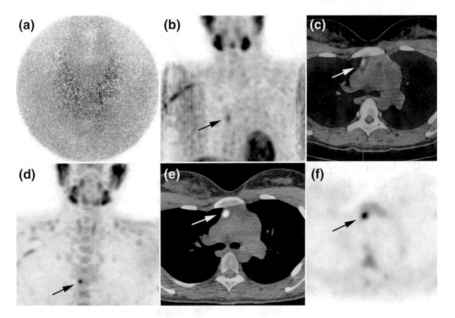

Fig. 5 Congenital PIII ectopia in the right thymus detected by PS and FCH PET/CT. Major ectopia of PIII (arrows) visualized on both SPECT/CT (**b** MIP image, **c** SPECT/CT fusion image) and FCH PET/CT (**d** subtraction MIP image, **e** PET/CT fusion image, **f** attenuation corrected PET image). The planar pinhole subtraction image (**a**) ruled out any additional cervical parathyroid lesion

18F-fluorocholine (FCH) is the PET tracer that is now the most investigated, but most studies are on primary hyperparathyroidism and little data exist for sHPT and tHPT (Figs. 3, 4 and 5).

Sensitivity of FCH-PET/CT is high in almost all recent reports in series of primary hyperparathyroidism [68–70], including in patients with previously negative or inconclusive ultrasound and/or sestamibi (usually dual-phase) imaging [71–73], or even reoperated patients [74]. Some studies, however, also showed that false-positive results can be induced by thyroid lesions or lymph nodes [70, 75]. Studies comparing 18F-choline to state-of-the-art 99mTc-sestamibi/iodine-123 subtraction scintigraphy are lacking and would be helpful to perform.

The potential role of contrast enhanced FCH PET/CT [76] as well as FCH PET/MR [77] would merit specific attention in complicated patients before reoperative surgery.

References

1. Ureña-Torres P, Vervloet M, Mazzaferro S, et al. Novel insights into parathyroid hormone: report of the parathyroid day in chronic kidney disease. Clin Kidney J. 2018;11:1–12.
2. Floege J, Kim J, Ireland E, et al. Serum iPTH, calcium and phosphate, and the risk of mortality in a European haemodialysis population. Nephrol Dial Transpl. 2011;26(6):1948–55.
3. Quarles LD. Role of FGF23 in vitamin D and phosphate metabolism: implications in chronic kidney disease. Exp Cell Res. 2012;318(9):1040–8.
4. Ganesh SK, Stack AG, Levin NW, Hulbert-Shearon T, Port FK. Association of elevated serum PO(4), Ca x PO(4) product, and parathyroid hormone with cardiac mortality risk in chronic hemodialysis patients. J Am Soc Nephrol. 2001;12(10):2131–8.
5. Tentori F, Blayney MJ, Albert JM, et al. Mortality risk for dialysis patients with different levels of serum calcium, phosphorus, and PTH: the dialysis outcomes and practice patterns study (DOPPS). Am J Kidney Dis. 2008;52(3):519–30.
6. Gutierrez OM, Januzzi JL, Isakova T, et al. Fibroblast growth factor 23 and left ventricular hypertrophy in chronic kidney disease. Circulation. 2009;119(19):2545–52.
7. K/DOQI clinical practice guidelines for bone metabolism and disease in chronic kidney disease. Am J Kidney Dis. 2003; 42(4 Suppl 3):S1–201.
8. KDIGO clinical practice guideline for the diagnosis, evaluation, prevention, and treatment of chronic kidney disease-mineral and bone disorder (CKD-MBD). Kidney Int Suppl. 2009; (113): S1–130.
9. Chertow GM, Block GA, Correa-Rotter R, et al. Effect of cinacalcet on cardiovascular disease in patients undergoing dialysis. N Engl J Med. 2012;367(26):2482–94.
10. Finnerty BM, Chan TW, Jones G, et al. Parathyroidectomy versus cinacalcet in the management of tertiary hyperparathyroidism: surgery improves renal transplant allograft survival. Surgery. 2019;165(1):129–34.
11. Dulfer RR, Koh EY, van der Plas WY, et al. Parathyroidectomy versus cinacalcet for tertiary hyperparathyroidism; a retrospective analysis. Langenbecks Arch Surg. 2019;404(1):71–9.
12. Chen L, Wang K, Yu S, et al. Long-term mortality after parathyroidectomy among chronic kidney disease patients with secondary hyperparathyroidism: a systematic review and meta-analysis. Ren Fail. 2016;38(7):1050–8.
13. Rodriguez-Ortiz ME, Pendon-Ruiz de Mier MV, Rodriguez M. Parathyroidectomy in dialysis patients: indications, methods, and consequences. Semin Dial. 2019.
14. Jofre R, Lopez Gomez JM, Menarguez J, et al. Parathyroidectomy: whom and when? Kidney Int Suppl. 2003;85:S97–100.

15. Madorin C, Owen RP, Fraser WD, et al. The surgical management of renal hyperparathyroidism. Eur Arch Otorhinolaryngol. 2012;269(6):1565–76.
16. Sharma J, Raggi P, Kutner N, et al. Improved long-term survival of dialysis patients after near-total parathyroidectomy. J Am Coll Surg. 2012; **214**(4):400–7; discussion 7–8.
17. Tominaga Y, Matsuoka S, Uno N. Surgical and medical treatment of secondary hyperparathyroidism in patients on continuous dialysis. World J Surg. 2009;33(11):2335–42.
18. Cruzado JM, Moreno P, Torregrosa JV, et al. A randomized study comparing parathyroidectomy with cinacalcet for treating hypercalcemia in kidney allograft recipients with hyperparathyroidism. J Am Soc Nephrol. 2016;27(8):2487–94.
19. van der Plas WY, Dulfer RR, Koh EY, et al. Safety and efficacy of subtotal or total parathyroidectomy for patients with secondary or tertiary hyperparathyroidism in four academic centers in the Netherlands. Langenbecks Arch Surg. 2018;403(8):999–1005.
20. Filho WA, van der Plas WY, Brescia MDG, et al. Quality of life after surgery in secondary hyperparathyroidism, comparing subtotal parathyroidectomy with total parathyroidectomy with immediate parathyroid autograft: Prospective randomized trial. Surgery. 2018;164(5):978–85.
21. Gagne ER, Urena P, Leite-Silva S, et al. Short- and long-term efficacy of total parathyroidectomy with immediate autografting compared with subtotal parathyroidectomy in hemodialysis patients. J Am Soc Nephrol. 1992;3(4):1008–17.
22. Kovacevic B, Ignjatovic M, Zivaljevic V, et al. Parathyroidectomy for the attainment of NKF-K/DOQI and KDIGO recommended values for bone and mineral metabolism in dialysis patients with uncontrollable secondary hyperparathyroidism. Langenbecks Arch Surg. 2012;397(3):413–20.
23. Mazzaferro S, Pasquali M, Farcomeni A, et al. Parathyroidectomy as a therapeutic tool for targeting the recommended NKF-K/DOQI ranges for serum calcium, phosphate and parathyroid hormone in dialysis patients. Nephrol Dial Transplant. 2008;23(7):2319–23.
24. Taterra D, Wong LM, Vikse J, et al. The prevalence and anatomy of parathyroid glands: a meta-analysis with implications for parathyroid surgery. Langenbecks Arch Surg. 2019;404(1):63–70.
25. Akerstrom G, Malmaeus J, Bergstrom R. Surgical anatomy of human parathyroid glands. Surgery. 1984;95(1):14–21.
26. Gwiasda J, Kaltenborn A, Muller JA, et al. Ultrasound-based scores as predictors for nodular hyperplasia in patients with secondary hyperparathyroidism: a prospective validation study. Langenbecks Arch Surg. 2017;402(2):295–301.
27. Vulpio C, Bossola M. Parathyroid ultrasonography in renal secondary hyperparathyroidism: an overlooked and useful procedure. Semin Dial. 2016;29(5):347–9.
28. Vulpio C, Bossola M, De Gaetano A, et al. Parathyroid gland ultrasound patterns and biochemical findings after one-year cinacalcet treatment for advanced secondary hyperparathyroidism. Ther Apher Dial. 2010;14(2):178–85.
29. Jeanguillaume C, Urena P, Hindie E, et al. Secondary hyperparathyroidism: detection with I-123-Tc-99m-Sestamibi subtraction scintigraphy versus US. Radiology. 1998;207(1):207–13.
30. Loftus KA, Anderson S, Mulloy AL, Terris DJ. Value of sestamibi scans in tertiary hyperparathyroidism. Laryngoscope. 2007;117(12):2135–8.
31. Andrade JS, Mangussi-Gomes JP, Rocha LA, et al. Localization of ectopic and supernumerary parathyroid glands in patients with secondary and tertiary hyperparathyroidism: surgical description and correlation with preoperative ultrasonography and Tc99m-Sestamibi scintigraphy. Braz J Otorhinolaryngol. 2014;80(1):29–34.
32. Karipineni F, Sahli Z, Somervell H, et al. Are preoperative sestamibi scans useful for identifying ectopic parathyroid glands in patients with expected multigland parathyroid disease? Surgery. 2018;163(1):35–41.

33. Vulpio C, Bossola M, De Gaetano A, et al. Usefulness of the combination of ultrasonography and 99mTc-sestamibi scintigraphy in the preoperative evaluation of uremic secondary hyperparathyroidism. Head Neck. 2010;32(9):1226–35.
34. Hindie E, Urena P, Jeanguillaume C, et al. Preoperative imaging of parathyroid glands with technetium-99m-labelled sestamibi and iodine-123 subtraction scanning in secondary hyperparathyroidism. Lancet. 1999;353(9171):2200–4.
35. Taieb D, Urena-Torres P, Zanotti-Fregonara P, et al. Parathyroid scintigraphy in renal hyperparathyroidism: the added diagnostic value of SPECT and SPECT/CT. Clin Nucl Med. 2013.
36. Taillefer R, Boucher Y, Potvin C, Lambert R. Detection and localization of parathyroid adenomas in patients with hyperparathyroidism using a single radionuclide imaging procedure with technetium-99m-sestamibi (double-phase study). J Nucl Med. 1992;33(10):1801–7.
37. Piga M, Bolasco P, Satta L, et al. Double phase parathyroid technetium-99m-MIBI scintigraphy to identify functional autonomy in secondary hyperparathyroidism. J Nucl Med. 1996;37(4):565–9.
38. Martin D, Rosen IB, Ichise M. Evaluation of single isotope technetium 99M-sestamibi in localization efficiency for hyperparathyroidism. Am J Surg. 1996;172(6):633–6.
39. Hindie E, Melliere D, Jeanguillaume C, chéhadé F, Galle P. Acquisition double-fenêtre 99mTcMIBI/123I vs 99mTc-MIBI seul dans l'hyperparathyroïdie primitive. XXXVe Colloque de Médecine Nucléaire. 1996.
40. Hindie E, Melliere D, Jeanguillaume C, Perlemuter L, Chehade F, Galle P. Parathyroid imaging using simultaneous double-window recording of technetium-99m-sestamibi and iodine-123. J Nucl Med. 1998;39(6):1100–5.
41. Caveny SA, Klingensmith WC 3rd, Martin WE, et al. Parathyroid imaging: the importance of dual-radiopharmaceutical simultaneous acquisition with 99mTc-sestamibi and 123I. J Nucl Med Technol. 2012;40(2):104–10.
42. Tunninen V, Varjo P, Schildt J, et al. Comparison of five parathyroid scintigraphic protocols. Int J Mol Imaging. 2013;2013:921260.
43. Klingensmith WC 3rd, Koo PJ, Summerlin A, et al. Parathyroid imaging: the importance of pinhole collimation with both single- and dual-tracer acquisition. J Nucl Med Technol. 2013;41(2):99–104.
44. Guerin C, Lowery A, Gabriel S, et al. Preoperative imaging for focused parathyroidectomy: making a good strategy even better. Eur J Endocrinol. 2015.
45. Krakauer M, Wieslander B, Myschetzky PS, et al. A prospective comparative study of parathyroid dual-phase scintigraphy, dual-isotope subtraction scintigraphy, 4D-CT, and ultrasonography in primary hyperparathyroidism. Clin Nucl Med. 2016;41(2):93–100.
46. Schalin-Jantti C, Ryhanen E, Heiskanen I, et al. Planar scintigraphy with 123I/99mTc-sestamibi, 99mTc-sestamibi SPECT/CT, 11C-methionine PET/CT, or selective venous sampling before reoperation of primary hyperparathyroidism? J Nucl Med. 2013;54(5):739–47.
47. Hindie E, Ugur O, Fuster D, et al. 2009 EANM parathyroid guidelines. Eur J Nucl Med Mol Imaging. 2009;36(7):1201–16.
48. Zhang L, Xing C, Shen C, et al. Diagnostic accuracy study of intraoperative and perioperative serum intact PTH level for successful parathyroidectomy in 501 secondary hyperparathyroidism patients. Sci Rep. 2016;6:26841.
49. Wetmore JB, Liu J, Do TP, et al. Changes in secondary hyperparathyroidism-related biochemical parameters and medication use following parathyroidectomy. Nephrol Dial Transplant. 2016;31(1):103–11.
50. Konturek A, Barczynski M, Stopa M, Nowak W. Subtotal parathyroidectomy for secondary renal hyperparathyroidism: a 20-year surgical outcome study. Langenbecks Arch Surg. 2016;401(7):965–74.

51. Nastos K, Constantinides V, Mizamtsidi M, Duncan N, Tolley N, Palazzo F. Morbidity in parathyroid surgery for renal disease is under reported: a comparison of outcomes with primary hyperparathyroidism. Ann R Coll Surg Engl. 2018;100(6):436–42.

52. Alkhalili E, Tasci Y, Aksoy E, et al. The utility of neck ultrasound and sestamibi scans in patients with secondary and tertiary hyperparathyroidism. World J Surg. 2015;39(3):701–5.

53. Dotzenrath C, Cupisti K, Goretzki E, et al. Operative treatment of renal autonomous hyperparathyroidism: cause of persistent or recurrent disease in 304 patients. Langenbecks Arch Surg. 2003;387(9–10):348–54.

54. Hindie E, Zanotti-Fregonara P, Tabarin A, et al. The role of radionuclide imaging in the surgical management of primary hyperparathyroidism. J Nucl Med. 2015;56(5):737–44.

55. Gasparri G, Camandona M, Bertoldo U, et al. The usefulness of preoperative dual-phase 99mTc MIBI-scintigraphy and IO-PTH assay in the treatment of secondary and tertiary hyperparathyroidism. Ann Surg. 2009;250(6):868–71.

56. de la Rosa A, Jimeno J, Membrilla E, Sancho JJ, Pereira JA, Sitges-Serra A. Usefulness of preoperative Tc-mibi parathyroid scintigraphy in secondary hyperparathyroidism. Langenbecks Arch Surg. 2008;393(1):21–4.

57. Torregrosa JV, Fernandez-Cruz L, Canalejo A, et al. (99m)Tc-sestamibi scintigraphy and cell cycle in parathyroid glands of secondary hyperparathyroidism. World J Surg. 2000;24(11):1386–90.

58. Fuster D, Torregrosa JV, Domenech B, et al. Dual-phase 99mTc-MIBI scintigraphy to assess calcimimetic effect in patients on haemodialysis with secondary hyperparathyroidism. Nucl Med Commun. 2009;30(11):890–4.

59. Fuster D, Ybarra J, Ortin J, et al. Role of pre-operative imaging using 99mTc-MIBI and neck ultrasound in patients with secondary hyperparathyroidism who are candidates for subtotal parathyroidectomy. Eur J Nucl Med Mol Imaging. 2006;33(4):467–73.

60. Taieb D, Urena-Torres P, Zanotti-Fregonara P, et al. Parathyroid scintigraphy in renal hyperparathyroidism: the added diagnostic value of SPECT and SPECT/CT. Clin Nucl Med. 2013;38(8):630–5.

61. Pitt SC, Panneerselvan R, Chen H, Sippel RS. Tertiary hyperparathyroidism: is less than a subtotal resection ever appropriate? A study of long-term outcomes. Surgery. 2009;146(6):1130–7.

62. Triponez F, Kebebew E, Dosseh D, et al. Less-than-subtotal parathyroidectomy increases the risk of persistent/recurrent hyperparathyroidism after parathyroidectomy in tertiary hyperparathyroidism after renal transplantation. Surgery. 2006; **140**(6): 990–7; discussion 7–9.

63. Hindie E, Zanotti-Fregonara P, Just PA, et al. Parathyroid scintigraphy findings in chronic kidney disease patients with recurrent hyperparathyroidism. Eur J Nucl Med Mol Imaging. 2010;37(3):623–34.

64. Madorin CA, Owen R, Coakley B, et al. Comparison of radiation exposure and cost between dynamic computed tomography and sestamibi scintigraphy for preoperative localization of parathyroid lesions. JAMA Surg. 2013;148(6):500–3.

65. Kluijfhout WP, Pasternak JD, Drake FT, et al. Use of PET tracers for parathyroid localization: a systematic review and meta-analysis. Langenbecks Arch Surg. 2016;401(7):925–35.

66. Treglia G, Piccardo A, Imperiale A, et al. Diagnostic performance of choline PET for detection of hyperfunctioning parathyroid glands in hyperparathyroidism: a systematic review and meta-analysis. Eur J Nucl Med Mol Imaging. 2019;46(3):751–65.

67. Broos WAM, van der Zant FM, Knol RJJ, Wondergem M. Choline PET/CT in parathyroid imaging: a systematic review. Nucl Med Commun. 2019;40(2):96–105.

68. Beheshti M, Hehenwarter L, Paymani Z, et al. (18)F-fluorocholine PET/CT in the assessment of primary hyperparathyroidism compared with (99m)Tc-MIBI or (99m)Tc-tetrofosmin SPECT/CT: a prospective dual-centre study in 100 patients. Eur J Nucl Med Mol Imaging. 2018;45(10):1762–71.

69. Huber GF, Hullner M, Schmid C, et al. Benefit of (18)F-fluorocholine PET imaging in parathyroid surgery. Eur Radiol. 2018;28(6):2700–7.

70. Thanseer N, Bhadada SK, Sood A, et al. Comparative effectiveness of ultrasonography, 99mTc-sestamibi, and 18F-fluorocholine PET/CT in detecting parathyroid adenomas in patients with primary hyperparathyroidism. Clin Nucl Med. 2017;42(12):e491–7.

71. Fischli S, Suter-Widmer I, Nguyen BT, et al. The significance of 18F-fluorocholine-PET/CT as localizing imaging technique in patients with primary hyperparathyroidism and negative conventional imaging. Front Endocrinol (Lausanne). 2017;8:380.

72. Grimaldi S, Young J, Kamenicky P, et al. Challenging pre-surgical localization of hyperfunctioning parathyroid glands in primary hyperparathyroidism: the added value of (18)F-fluorocholine PET/CT. Eur J Nucl Med Mol Imaging. 2018;45(10):1772–80.

73. Quak E, Blanchard D, Houdu B, et al. F18-choline PET/CT guided surgery in primary hyperparathyroidism when ultrasound and MIBI SPECT/CT are negative or inconclusive: the APACH1 study. Eur J Nucl Med Mol Imaging. 2018;45(4):658–66.

74. Amadou C, Bera G, Ezziane M, et al. 18F-fluorocholine PET/CT and parathyroid 4D computed tomography for primary hyperparathyroidism: the challenge of reoperative patients. World J Surg. 2019.

75. Michaud L, Balogova S, Burgess A, et al. A pilot comparison of 18F-fluorocholine PET/CT, ultrasonography and 123I/99mTc-sestaMIBI dual-phase dual-isotope scintigraphy in the preoperative localization of hyperfunctioning parathyroid glands in primary or secondary hyperparathyroidism: influence of thyroid anomalies. Medicine (Baltimore). 2015;94(41):e1701.

76. Piccardo A, Trimboli P, Rutigliani M, et al. Additional value of integrated (18)F-choline PET/4D contrast-enhanced CT in the localization of hyperfunctioning parathyroid glands and correlation with molecular profile. Eur J Nucl Med Mol Imaging. 2019;46(3):766–75.

77. Kluijfhout WP, Pasternak JD, Beninato T, et al. Diagnostic performance of computed tomography for parathyroid adenoma localization; a systematic review and meta-analysis. Eur J Radiol. 2017;88:117–28.

PTH Receptors and Skeletal Resistance to PTH Action

Jordi Bover, Pablo A. Ureña-Torres, Pieter Evenepoel, Maria Jesús Lloret, Lluis Guirado and Mariano Rodríguez

Introduction

Chronic kidney disease (CKD) is an important global health problem, involving about 10% of the population worldwide and entailing high cardiovascular and mortality risks [1, 2]. CKD-mineral and bone disorder (CKD-MBD) is one of the many complications associated with CKD and represents a *systemic* disorder manifested by either one or a combination of: (a) abnormalities of calcium (Ca), phosphate (P), parathyroid hormone (PTH), or vitamin D metabolism; (b) abnormalities in bone turnover, mineralization, volume, linear growth, or strength (formerly known as renal osteodystrophy); and (c) vascular or other soft tissue calcifications [3–5]. Consequently, renal osteodystrophy is currently considered one measure of the skeletal component of CKD-MBD, which is quantifiable by bone histomorphometry, and recent knowledge indicates bone to be an endocrine organ at the heart of metabolic and cardiovascular complications of CKD [6].

Increased PTH levels [classically referred to as secondary hyperparathyroidism (SHPT)] are an integral component of the CKD-MBD syndrome and if they remain uncontrolled, they will worsen the laboratory abnormalities of CKD-MBD (e.g., calcium and phosphate levels), the bone structure (high-turnover bone disease), and cardiovascular parameters (e.g., vascular calcification)

J. Bover (✉) · M. J. Lloret · L. Guirado
Fundació Puigvert, Department of Nephrology, IIB Sant Pau, RedinRen, C. Cartagena 340, 08025 Barcelona, Catalonia, Spain
e-mail: jbover@fundacio-puigvert.es

P.A. Ureña-Torres
Department of Dialysis, AURA Nord Saint Ouen, Department of Renal Physiology, Necker Hospital, University of Paris Descartes, Paris, France

P. Evenepoel
University Hospitals Leuven, Louvain, Belgium

M. Rodríguez
Servicio Nefrología, Hospital Universitario Reina Sofía, IMIBIC, UCO, Córdoba, Spain

© Springer Nature Switzerland AG 2020
A. Covic et al. (eds.), *Parathyroid Glands in Chronic Kidney Disease*,
https://doi.org/10.1007/978-3-030-43769-5_4

[7–9]. Moreover, PTH has also classically been considered a "uremic toxin" [10] since the effect of PTH appears not to be limited to bone [11, 12]. Indeed SHPT has been claimed to contribute to many "off-target" extraskeletal clinical manifestations frequently present in CKD [11, 12]. For instance, PTH produces an increase in cytosolic "intracellular calcium" in many different cell types [13, 14] and this may be a common pathway that explains the relationship of PTH with many other systemic effects such as cognitive decline, cachexia, peripheral neuropathy, increasing osmotic fragility of erythrocytes, abnormalities of the immune system, muscular dysfunction and wasting, decreased testosterone and increased prolactin serum levels, carbohydrate intolerance and lipid abnormalities, renin-angiotensin-aldosterone system stimulation, myocardial dysfunction, and cardiac hypertrophy and fibrosis [11, 12, 15–17]. The improvement of some of these deleterious outcomes (e.g., left ventricular hypertrophy) following parathyroidectomy (PTX) supports the hypothesis of a causal link with PTH, although evidence of a direct role is still lacking [12, 18]. The above-mentioned toxic effects of PTH may explain the association of SHPT with CKD progression and atheromatous and non-atheromatous cardiovascular disease, as well as with all-cause and/or cardiovascular morbidity and mortality [19–23].

SHPT is classically considered a common, serious, and progressive complication of CKD. In the United States, the estimated prevalence of SHPT in CKD patients ranges from 2 to nearly 5 million individuals, with 30–50% of dialysis patients being affected with SHPT [24]. However, very low or relatively low PTH levels (which are associated with adynamic bone disease) are also considered an important contributory factor to the high morbidity and mortality in CKD patients [20, 25]. An increased risk of fractures and cardiovascular calcifications have been related to low PTH levels and is attributable to the inability of bone to buffer an excess of Ca and P loading [26]. Therefore, it is not surprising that associations between mortality and PTH are recognized to be complex, except at both extremes (high and low) of serum PTH levels [27]. Similarly, cohort studies have clearly indicated that only extreme levels are able to predict with acceptable sensitivity/ specificity the bone turnover status [from adynamic bone disease (low-turnover) to osteitis fibrosa (high-turnover bone disease) [4, 28]. Although PTH is a crucial determinant of bone remodeling [12], in uremic conditions it does not offer information on bone properties and strength, similarly to most bone markers [12, 29, 30]. Beyond the CKD population, investigations of cohorts of primarily cardiology patients have confirmed the independent association between high PTH levels, cardiovascular events, and mortality (including sudden cardiac death) [31–33].

Pathophysiology of Secondary Hyperparathyroidism

It is well known that progressive loss of kidney function leads to an increased P load (retention) [34, 35], increased fibroblast growth factor 23 (FGF23) and decreased α-klotho [36–38], and decreased synthesis and increased catabolism of calcitriol (1,25-dihydroxyvitamin D; active vitamin D), among many other metabolic derangements [15, 39]. All these factors, extensively reviewed elsewhere [15, 40, 41], involve various closely interacting mechanisms, including the down-regulation of Ca-sensing, vitamin D, and FGF23 receptors, and contribute in increasing the synthesis and secretion of PTH by the parathyroid glands as well as the proliferation (polyclonal and/or monoclonal) of parathyroid cells. It is well known that hyperplasia of the parathyroid glands starts to develop during the very early stages of CKD [11, 15, 42, 43].

Although it is currently known that P can both directly and indirectly induce SHPT in patients with CKD [44–46], it is widely accepted that Ca is the most important regulator of parathyroid gland function [12]. In order to correct *hypocalcemia*, rapid release of stored PTH is necessary, with increased synthesis and, eventually, parathyroid cell proliferation if required to produce the necessary amount of PTH to correct Ca. Thus, most of the previously mentioned mechanisms (e.g., P retention, decreased calcitriol production) share in common the capability to lead to secondary multifactorial hypocalcemia and hence induce SHPT. In the parathyroid cell, the transmembrane Ca-sensing receptor (CaSR), the complex FGFR1-klotho receptor complex, and the nuclear parathyroid vitamin D receptor (VDR) are down-regulated, resulting in increased PTH synthesis and secretion as well as parathyroid cell proliferation [47, 48]. It is beyond the scope of this review to analyze the complex interrelationships among all these pathophysiologic factors leading to SHPT. Rather, the focus will be on analysis of the importance of skeletal resistance to the action of PTH in the pathogenesis of SHPT and, on the other hand, the development of adynamic bone disease, since this remains greatly underappreciated by the nephrology community.

Skeletal Resistance to PTH Action

"Skeletal" resistance to the action of PTH in CKD (also known as calcemic resistance to PTH or PTH resistance) is an old concept [49], recently recognized as "hyporesponsiveness" to PTH [27, 50]. In fact, both bone and renal responses to the action of PTH are progressively impaired in CKD [27] and the term "hyporesponsiveness" may be more appropriate because the response to PTH is blunted but not completely absent [27].

A decreased calcemic response to PTH was first described by J. M. Evanson in 1966 [49] when he reported the calcemic response to an infusion of crude parathyroid *extract* (1 U/kg/h over 10 h) to be significantly lower in 12 hypocalcemic patients with CKD than in normal subjects or patients with primary hyperparathyroidism [49]. He postulated that vitamin D is necessary for the action of PTH on bone, since a decreased calcemic response was also observed in hypocalcemic patients with steatorrhea or rickets [49]. Subsequently, Massry et al. observed that the calcemic response to a parathyroid *extract* (2 IU/kg over 8 h) in thyroparathyroidectomized (T-PTX) dogs, before and after the induction of uremia by bilateral ureteral ligation (BUL) or by bilateral nephrectomy, was markedly impaired, but that the impairment was more severe one day after nephrectomy [51]. They also observed that the calcemic response after 2 or 3 days of BUL was similar to that seen at one day after nephrectomy and that calcitriol partially restored the calcemic response to PTH [51]. The authors concluded that a deficiency of calcitriol was at least partly responsible for the skeletal resistance to the calcemic action of PTH in the presence of uremia and that uremia, per se, could also have contributed to this phenomenon. In addition, it was observed that the calcemic response to PTH was lower in *patients* with moderate and advanced CKD (including hemodialysis and renal transplant patients) than in normal healthy subjects [52]. This reduced calcemic response was not related to the initial levels of serum Ca, P, or PTH and was not reversed by hemodialysis [52].

Llach et al. also noted a decreased calcemic response to *endogenous* PTH and an altered divalent ion metabolism in *patients* with early CKD [53, 54]. For instance, they described delayed recovery from ethylene diamine tetra-acetic acid (EDTA)-induced hypocalcemia in these patients as compared with normal subjects, despite higher serum PTH levels in the CKD group [53]. Such observations indicated that the impaired calcemic response to PTH appears early in the course of CKD and that a direct consequence is a continuous requirement for a greater concentration of circulating PTH in order to maintain a normal Ca homeostasis in affected patients. Ever since the study by Albright et al. [55] it has been hypothesized that P retention and reciprocal blood Ca lowering in CKD patients might cause parathyroid hyperplasia and renal osteitis fibrosa. With the formulation of the "trade-off" hypothesis by Bricker and Slatopolsky [34, 56–58], the reduction in the level of serum Ca in CKD was considered to be the main driver of increased synthesis and secretion of PTH, as well as parathyroid hyperplasia. However, the presence of skeletal resistance to PTH in CKD provides a usually forgotten additional mechanism in the pathogenesis of hypocalcemia and SHPT in CKD [15, 59, 60]. The appearance of skeletal resistance to the action of PTH *early* in the course of renal failure would induce hypocalcemia, which in turn would stimulate the parathyroid glands, resulting in continuously increased secretion of the hormone and hyperplasia. At the other extreme, the *late* appearance of detectable hypocalcemia in advanced stages of CKD [61] clearly represents the final failure of PTH to restore Ca levels to normal, and the maximal clinical expression of hyporesponsiveness to PTH.

Factors Linked to Impaired Calcemic Response to PTH (See Table 1)

Decreased Levels of Calcitriol

Since the earliest work in this field it was considered that vitamin D appears to be necessary for the proper action of PTH on bone [49]. Later, it was demonstrated that the administration of calcitriol restored, at least partially, the blunted calcemic response to PTH in experimental animals (rats and dogs) [51, 62, 63] leading to the conclusion that this impaired calcemic response to PTH is related to the decreased calcitriol levels observed in early CKD. Also, in *patients* with early CKD, daily administration of 0.5 µg of calcitriol for 6 weeks improved the calcemic response to PTH [54]. Finally, studies in experimental animals also exhibited complete correction of the calcemic response to PTH after the administration of calcitriol [$1,25(OH)_2D_3$] together with $24,25(OH)_2D_3$ [64]. Consequently, although an adequate mechanistic explanation for these observations is still lacking, it seems clear that reduced serum vitamin D levels play a role in the impaired calcemic response to PTH, and that vitamin D could enhance the action of PTH on bone. However, other investigators did not confirm this beneficial effect of calcitriol on the calcemic response to PTH [62, 65]. There is also no scientific evidence demonstrating that the correction of native vitamin D deficiency (25OHD < 15 ng/ml), which is often the case in CKD, by restoring serum 25OHD levels, would improve the calcemic response to PTH.

Phosphate Retention

It is also well known that P retention significantly decreases the calcemic response to PTH in CKD [63, 66]. Somerville and Kaye reinfused urine into T-PTX rats, inducing *acute* uremia in the presence of normal kidneys, and observed that the calcemic response to PTH after 5 h of PTH extract infusion was clearly blunted. Removal of P by treating urine with zirconium oxide completely restored the calcemic response to PTH [66]. Moreover, other groups of T-PTX rats given PTH extract were infused with an electrolyte solution containing varying amounts of P up to a maximum similar to the amount that a urine-infused rat would receive. A highly significant inverse relationship was found between the dose of P infused with the electrolyte solution and the measured calcemic response to PTH [66]. Since P and calcitriol are also closely interrelated (P inhibits the synthesis of calcitriol), it could not be excluded that at least some of these observations might be mediated indirectly by inhibition of calcitriol. Thus, using a different model, Rodriguez et al. [63] demonstrated that rats with CKD fed with a low-P diet exhibited an improvement in the calcemic response during a constant 48-h infusion of 1–34 rat PTH with an ALZET® pump; moreover, rats with either moderate or advanced CKD had an impaired calcemic response to PTH and low levels of calcitriol. The low-P diet enhanced the calcemic response to PTH in both groups of rats, but only those with moderate CKD had a significant increment in calcitriol levels. Thus, with moderate CKD, P restriction improved the calcemic response to PTH, and this effect could be due to higher levels of calcitriol. However, in advanced CKD, the calcemic response to PTH improved with P restriction *independently* of calcitriol. As a matter of fact, we observed that the negative effect of P retention on the calcemic response to PTH may be far superior to the effect of calcitriol deficiency in rats with CKD [67, 68] (See Fig. 1).

Improvement of the calcemic response to a standardized infusion of PTH after P restriction has also been demonstrated in *patients* with mild CKD [69]. Interestingly, in rats with normal renal function that received a high-P diet, the calcemic response to PTH was reduced in the absence of any change in serum P levels; this indicates that the diet itself was responsible for the reduction in response. This is an issue that should be taken into consideration currently, given the lack of a clear recommendation on whether dietary P restriction should be applied in CKD stages 2–3. The intrinsic mechanism that leads to a P-induced decrease in the calcemic response to PTH is not completely known but, in addition to the effect of P on calcitriol levels, the ambient P concentration in bone may affect the amount of exchangeable Ca that can be mobilized by PTH [62, 70].

All of the above experiments were done before the discovery of FGF23, and to date the possibility that high FGF23 (which may act on osteoblasts) may reduce the calcemic effect of PTH on bone has not been excluded. It could be that high FGF23 either directly or indirectly (via calcitriol suppression, Dkk1 stimulation or sclerostin) interferes with PTH-mediated Ca efflux from bone. Moreover, multiple binding sites for Ca^{2+} and PO_4^{3-} ions have been described at the CaSR [71]. While Ca^{2+} ions stabilize its active state, PO_4^{3-} ions reinforce the *inactive* conformation of the CaSR, thus contributing to increased PTH secretion [71]. A similar inactivating effect of P on the bone CaSR could also be involved in such reduced calcemic response to PTH in CKD.

Although both P restriction and calcitriol supplementation *improve* the calcemic response to PTH, they do not seem to completely restore it, either alone or together. Conversely, in PTX dogs or rats [63, 65, 72], the removal of circulating PTH corrects the calcemic response to PTH despite the presence of hyperphosphatemia and low calcitriol levels.

Down-Regulation of PTH Receptors

The aforementioned findings suggested that high levels of endogenous PTH levels in PTX uremic animals could have desensitized the skeleton to the administration of exogenous PTH [65, 73]. The role of down-regulation of PTH bone receptors by high PTH levels was established after the observation that the removal of PTH seemed to restore the responsiveness to its receptors. Likewise, it was described in isolated perfused bones from uremic dogs with acute or chronic renal failure that the release of cyclic adenosine monophosphate (cAMP) was blunted in response to PTH, whereas it was restored by T-PTX [74, 75]. Although PTX corrected the calcemic response to PTH in experimental uremia, we noted that holding PTH levels in the normal range in rats with CKD fed with a low-P diet did *not* correct the calcemic response to PTH [72]. Thus, uremic rats with normal PTH levels, achieved with partial PTX, still showed a 50% decrease in the calcemic response to PTH as compared with normal rats [72]. This is consistent with clinical studies showing that subtotal PTX resulted in almost normal PTH levels but did not enhance the calcemic response to PTH [52]. Similarly, PTX improved the calcemic response to PTH not only in animals with CKD but also in sham-operated rats [72]. Therefore, PTH-induced down-regulation of PTH receptors appeared not to be the sole explanation for the decrease in the calcemic response to PTH in CKD. It was hypothesized that the significant improvement in the calcemic response to PTH after PTX could be due to a phenomenon of hypersensitization following hormone depletion, as described for other hormonal systems, among other potential explanations affecting the exchangeable Ca pool in bone described elsewhere [72, 76].

All of these findings do not exclude down-regulation of PTH receptors as a potential cause of the decreased calcemic response to PTH [77]. Thus, the cloning of a ubiquitous PTH receptor (PTHR) gene—a common receptor for both PTH and PTH-related peptide (PTHrP) [78, 79]—has allowed demonstration that the PTH1R (PTHR-1) is not only widely distributed in tissues [80] but also down-regulated in uremic kidneys, epiphyseal cartilage growth plates, and osteoblasts, at least at the transcription level [81–84]. Human data are less consistent, with some investigators demonstrating decreased expression [85] while others have recently reported increased expression [86]. Methodological issues and variation in the characteristics of the studied populations may explain this apparent discrepancy [27].

The finding of down-regulation of the PTH1R mRNA in bone tissue and not in the liver or heart suggested that PTH1R expression is regulated in a cell-specific manner regardless of the uremic state [87]. It is likely, however, that factors other than the increased PTH levels down-regulate this receptor [82, 87]. Thus, Ureña et al. showed the expression of PTH1R mRNA to be decreased in kidneys from both rats with CKD and rats with CKD that were subjected to PTX [87]. Since PTX did not restore the expression of PTH1R mRNA, elevation of PTH levels would not be necessary to induce its down-regulation in CKD. Their data also demonstrated that neither an increase in plasma PTH and P nor a decrease in plasma Ca is important in renal PTH1R down-regulation during CKD, and that it is also unlikely that an increase in the locally produced renal PTHrP could down-regulate its own receptor. However, other authors observed *increased* expression of PTH1R mRNA after PTX, but controls were not available [83].

Although the mechanisms responsible for the putative desensitization or down-regulation of PTH1R in CKD remain very poorly defined, several studies have implicated several uremic factors and C-terminal PTH fragments (see below). The available information on PTH1R regulation is very limited and even contradictory, and beyond the scope of this review [88–91].

Uremia

Importantly, in experimental rats with CKD we observed a significant decrease in the calcemic response to a 48-h rat 1–34 PTH infusion despite the presence of normal serum Ca, P, calcitriol, and PTH levels. This finding suggests that factors intrinsic to uremia may, per se, impair the calcemic response to PTH [72]. These data were subsequently confirmed in a different model when Berdud et al. [92] observed that maintenance of *normal* PTH levels in uremic PTX rats by constant infusion of PTH did not correct the impaired calcemic response to PTH.

The presence of unknown uremic factors, beyond P, that are potentially responsible for the decreased calcemic response to PTH in CKD had already been postulated previously [52]. Similarly, Wills and Jenkins had also shown that serum from uremic patients inhibited PTH-induced bone resorption in an in vitro model, whereas serum obtained after dialysis did not [93]. Low molecular weight inhibitors of osteoblast mitogenesis in uremic plasma were described [94], and subsequent experimental studies pointed towards different uremic toxins [95] triggering oxidative stress, such as indoxyl sulfate (IS) and *p*-cresyl sulfate (PCS) [96, 97] and/or inflammatory bioactive oxidized low-density lipoproteins [98]. Increased oxidative stress and low-degree inflammation are common conditions in CKD, and thus they may be not only causal but also common pathways (e.g., P retention or calcitriol deficiency is also associated with oxidative stress and inflammation) linking CKD and PTH hyporesponsiveness [27]. In vitro studies [99] have shown that the uremic toxin IS inhibits not only osteoblast but also osteoclast differentiation and function, and that these effects are enhanced in the presence of high P concentrations. In vivo studies [100] have also shown that the administration of the oral charcoal adsorbent AST-120 prevented low-turnover bone in uremic rats. Nii-Kono et al. [96] further showed that IS induces a state of PTH resistance, consisting in a reduction of PTH-induced cAMP and PTHR gene expression, and decreases the viability of osteoblasts maintained in culture. These authors also demonstrated that free radical production in osteoblasts increases in relation to the concentration of IS added [96]. Furthermore, their results suggested that IS is taken up by osteoblasts via the organic anion transporter-3, augmenting oxidative stress to impair osteoblast function and down-regulate PTH1R expression [96]. On the other hand, contradictory results have recently been reported by Barreto et al. [101], who showed a *positive* association of serum IS with osteoblast surface and bone formation rate in 49 CKD stage 2–3 patients (36 ± 17 ml/min/1.73 m^2); however, this study may have been largely underpowered to address this question. Although the temporal sequence is unknown, it is possible that early accumulation of uremic toxins induces skeletal PTH hyporesponsiveness and therefore contributes to the initial adaptive increase in PTH (initial biochemical SHPT) in order to normalize the important serum Ca (and P) levels. At a certain point, the progressive increase in serum PTH levels could then override the described direct inhibitory effects of IS on bone turnover [39]. Finally, uremic toxins may also stimulate PTH secretion indirectly by decreasing calcitriol synthesis and binding to DNA vitamin D response elements [102, 103], inducing resistance to the inhibitory action of calcitriol.

PTH Abnormal Metabolism and Fragments in CKD

An increased rate of PTH secretion is primarily responsible for high plasma levels of PTH in CKD. However, evidence demonstrates that the kidneys play an important role in the degradation of PTH and that, in patients with CKD, the metabolic clearance of PTH, like that of other peptide hormones, is reduced.

PTH is a hormone actively secreted mainly by chief cells of the parathyroid gland as a single-chain polypeptide containing 84 amino acids (1–84 PTH) [104, 105]. The physiological role of the increased number of parathyroid oxyphil cells in CKD or the chief-to-oxyphil transdifferentiation is still largely unknown [106, 107]. As mentioned previously, PTH increases serum Ca by activation of the PTH1R, which is mainly present in bone and kidney but is also found in a variety of tissues not regarded as classic PTH targets. This explains the widespread effects of PTH and illustrates why PTH is considered to be a clinically relevant uremic toxin, at least in patients with advanced CKD [11].

The amino-terminal extreme of PTH is required for activation of adenyl-cyclase. The PTH1R, coupled to G-proteins, is activated equivalently by 1–84 PTH, amino-terminal PTH, and PTHrP.

PTH is physiologically released in episodic secretory bursts that are superimposed on a basal, tonic mode of secretion [108], and this pulsatile secretion may determine the balance between its catabolic and anabolic effects on the skeleton [109, 110]. Such pulsatility has been detected in both normal subjects and patients with CKD [108, 111]. Despite the pulsatile character of PTH release, intact PTH levels were found to be continuously maintained within the normal range in a control group and in CKD patients with normal parathyroid function whereas in CKD patients with SHPT, PTH changes were restricted within a level of hyperparathyroidism [111].

Secreted 1–84 PTH is degraded rapidly (half-life of approximately 2–4 min) to amino-terminal and carboxy-terminal fragments [112]. The amino-terminal residues bind to the PTH1R, activate cellular responses, and mimic all the Ca-regulating actions of PTH in animals [113]. The carboxy-terminal fragment of PTH seems to be essential for hormone processing (efficient transport across the endoplasmic reticulum) and secretion [114]. Although 1–84 PTH is the main source of secreted PTH, it is also known that the gland can secrete carboxy-terminal fragments and that the relative secretion of these fragments increases or decreases in the presence of hypercalcemia or hypocalcemia, respectively [115, 116]. Studies have shown that preferential secretion of carboxy-terminal fragments may not occur in primary hyperparathyroidism as it does in other hypercalcemic states [117], and that some subpopulations of parathyroid cells from hyperplastic or adenomatous glands can secrete in vitro more amino-terminal fragments than 1–84 PTH [118].

Because of the shorter half-lives of both 1–84 PTH and amino-terminal fragments, the carboxy-terminal fragments become the predominating PTH peptide in the circulation. The parent peptide is rapidly degraded in the peripheral tissues, particularly in the kidneys and the liver [11, 112, 119]. The liver has great capacity to degrade the peptide, but it may not play an important role in the degradation of fragments [120]. By contrast, the kidney can extract and degrade the complete molecule and its fragments [121], at least partially via the action of cathepsin D [122]. Thus, impairment of renal function causes accumulation of carboxy-terminal fragments, and although amino-terminal fragments are also produced by cleavage of 1–84 PTH (i.e., by Kupffer cells), they are rapidly degraded, unlike the corresponding carboxy-terminal fragments [11].

As mentioned above, carboxy-terminal fragments are mainly catabolized in the kidney, and the degradation process involves solely glomerular filtration and tubular reabsorption, whereas the amino-terminal fragment undergoes both tubular reabsorption and peritubular uptake, like 1–84 PTH [112]. These pathways of PTH metabolism are altered in the presence of CKD, and renal excretion of PTH and its fragments (mainly carboxy-terminal) is decreased [112, 123]. Therefore, such alterations in PTH metabolism also partially account for the elevated PTH levels observed in CKD.

Although PTH measurement with the current immunoradiometric (IRMA) and immunochemiluminescence assays directed to the so-called *intact* PTH (the most widely implemented worldwide) has significantly improved clinical management, several fragments still affect the measurement and interpretation of these second-generation *intact* PTH assays. Thus, it is now well known that there are non-(1–84)-PTH truncated fragments in the circulation (such as 7–84 PTH) which, in addition to 1–84 PTH, are measured by most IRMA intact PTH assays, giving erroneously high PTH values [27, 124, 125]. This fact is especially important now that many different (automated and non-automated) *non-standardized* intact PTH kits are available on the market, using different antibodies and without a common calibrator [11, 27, 126–129]. Consequently, there is wide variability among commercially available intact PTH assays [128]. Third-generation assays (measuring the so-called "whole" or "bioactive" PTH) seem to detect only the biologically active 1–84 PTH molecule because the detection antibody is more specific for the first four amino acids at the amino-terminal end [130, 131]. While these new-generation "whole PTH" assays do not interact with 7–84 PTH fragments, they seem to measure, in addition to 1–84 PTH, a post-translational form called amino-PTH [132]. In any case, "intact" and "whole" PTH assays appear to be of similar clinical value for the diagnosis of SHPT and the follow-up of CKD-MBD, and "whole"/"bio-intact" PTH measurement is not yet fully recommended in any guideline [4].

The recent description of *non-active* oxidized-PTH adds complexity to the clinical interpretation of PTH values [112, 133–136], and it has recently been debated whether the increased mortality risk associated with PTH might actually reflect an oxidative stress-related mortality [19, 112, 135]. Whereas it is widely accepted that PTH measurement (especially *trends*) is an appropriate marker of *parathyroid* activity, PTH is only indirectly and weakly associated with bone dynamics [137]. Therefore, over the last decade there has been increased controversy over the validity of PTH as a surrogate marker of CKD-MBD and/or bone turnover

[137, 138], as well as for the definition of optimal PTH targets in both non-dialysis and dialysis CKD patients [4, 139].

Furthermore, regarding the importance of these abnormalities in the metabolism of PTH for the calcemic response to PTH, it has been reported that, in PTX rats fed a calcium-deficient diet, 7–84 PTH was not only biologically inactive but also had *antagonistic* effects on the PTHR in kidney and bone [130]. In these animals, plasma Ca was increased 2 h after 1–84 PTH treatment, while 7–84 PTH had no effect. However, when 1–84 PTH and 7–84 PTH were given simultaneously in a 1:1 molar ratio, the calcemic response to 1–84 PTH was decreased by 94%. Moreover, the administration of 1–84 PTH increased the renal fractional excretion of P in normal rats. However, when 1–84 PTH and 7–84 PTH were given simultaneously, the 7–84 PTH decreased the phosphaturic response by 50.2%. Finally, in surgically excised parathyroid glands from six uremic patients, the authors found that 44.1% of the total intracellular PTH was the non-PTH (1–84), most likely PTH 7–84. They concluded that in patients with CKD, the presence of high circulating levels of non-1–84 PTH fragments detected by the "intact" assay and the antagonistic effects of 7–84 PTH on the biological activity of 1–84 PTH explain the need for higher levels of "intact" PTH to prevent adynamic bone disease and provide a novel mechanism for skeletal resistance to PTH in uremia [130].

In addition to the "classic" PTH1R, it is currently accepted that a carboxy-terminal PTHR (PTH4R or PTHR-C) may mediate these different actions [140–142]. Increasing evidence indicates that the C-terminal PTH fragments, by binding and competing with 1–84 PTH for the PTH1R or by binding to the PTHR-C, exert these different/opposite biological effects as compared to 1–84 PTH [11, 27, 130, 141, 143–145]. Actually, it has been shown that the effects of 7–84 PTH on 1–84 PTH secretion and on plasma Ca levels are not associated with changes in PTH, PTH1R, CaSR, and PTHrP gene expression in rat parathyroid glands [145], and it has been hypothesized that PTH 7–84 regulates PTH secretion via an autocrine/paracrine regulatory mechanism [145]. The biological significance of this system may relate to the fact that during hypercalcemia the PTHR-C may help to maintain normal bone formation when the carboxy-terminal fragments exceed those of 1–84 PTH. Therefore, it has been postulated that the ratio of 1–84 PTH (or amino-terminal PTH) to carboxy-terminal PTH, which would be equivalent to the opposite effects of PTH1R/PTHR-C receptor activation, may be important in understanding not only the changes in the parathyroid gland but also the bone activity observed in CKD patients [11]. Moreover, the increased production of large carboxy-terminal PTH fragments by parathyroid glands during hypercalcemia, mentioned earlier, may help to restore Ca by inhibition of bone resorption [11, 115]. This relative increase in C-terminal fragments has been demonstrated in hemodialysis patients exposed to low and high Ca concentrations in the dialysis bath [116].

Other PTH receptors (PTH2R and PTH3R) have also been described but their effects in humans and in CKD are largely unknown [12, 146, 147]. PTH2R is not expressed in renal tubules and bone and is not activated by PTHrP. Like PTH1R,

PTH2R responds to PTH with generation of cAMP and an increase in intracellular calcium.

Additional information on PTH metabolism and signaling, both in health and in CKD and including classic and non-classic target organs for PTH, may be found in recent review papers [11, 27].

Downstream Competing Signals, Local or Systemic Factors

It is possible that the downstream effects of PTH may be offset by associated competing and/or inhibitory endocrine or paracrine signals, mediated by, for example, FGF23, klotho, calcitonin, osteoprotegerin, bone morphogenetic proteins, Wnt antagonists, and insulin-like growth factors, in addition to local environmental factors (i.e., inflammation, cytokines, oxidative stress, acid-base disturbances, and Ca, P, magnesium, and aluminum concentrations) [27, 39].

Thus, a recent study demonstrated that a recombinant human *klotho* protein interacted with human PTH1R to inhibit the binding of human PTH in *renal* tubular cells. It also inhibited the PTH-induced 1-α-hydroxylase expression by tubular cells both in vitro and in vivo [148]. These results suggest that free klotho mediates the FGF23-induced inhibition of calcitriol synthesis [148], and it has been hypothesized that as long as PTH underlies basal production of calcitriol, free klotho mediates, at least in part, the decrease in calcitriol levels in response to FGF23 by impairing PTH signaling [148].

The role of endogenous *calcitonin* production by thyroid C cells in the pathogenesis of SHPT—in general, in the protection against hypercalcemia, and in the decreased calcemic response to PTH in CKD—has also been analyzed [149–154]. It has been shown that in the absence of calcitonin, the calcemic response to PTH increased in rats regardless of whether they had CKD or not. In the presence of SHPT and hypercalcemia, calcitonin was an important modifier of the calcemic response to PTH, especially in animals with CKD [149, 151].

There is scarce information about a potential role of *osteoprotegerin* (OPG, a potent osteoclast activation inhibitor) in the CKD-MBD complex. Since skeletal resistance to PTH appears as an anti-calcemic effect against exogenous PTH load in the physiological aspect, and as the discrepancy between serum PTH level and bone turnover in the morphological aspect, OPG has been postulated to be a common pathogenic mediator of both high- and low-bone turnover diseases [155, 156]. Thus, the high circulating OPG levels found in CKD [156] may promote skeletal resistance to PTH through suppression of osteo*clasto*genesis [155, 157].

Importantly, *Wnt antagonists* such as *sclerostin*, the product of the SOST gene and mainly produced by osteocytes, was originally believed to be a non-classic BMP antagonist [158]. Sclerostin has now been identified as a soluble inhibitor of the Wnt signaling pathway via binding to LRP5/6 receptors [159, 160], and hence it may lead to decreased bone formation by inhibiting osteo*blasto*genesis (in contrast to OPG). Sclerostin may also play a role in the mediation of systemic and local factors such as calcitriol, PTH, glucocorticoids, and tumor necrosis factor-α [161]. Circulating sclerostin levels increase with age and with declining renal function [161–163] and are also increased in diabetic patients independently of gender and age [164]. Levels decrease rapidly after renal transplantation [165, 166]. Nevertheless, it remains a matter of debate to what extent circulating sclerostin levels reflect bone expression and affect local signaling, since discrepant findings have been described [167]. Increased osteocytic sclerostin expression has indeed been observed in early-stage CKD despite still normal serum PTH levels [168], and the increase persists in dialysis patients, although to a lesser extent, despite elevated PTH levels [169].

Sclerostin and the related Dickkopf-1 (Dkk1) or secreted frizzled-related protein 4 (sFRP4) have been postulated to be potentially important mediators of the development of adynamic bone disease [12, 39, 97, 170] and/or skeletal resistance to the action of PTH [39, 97, 170]. A new paradigm is evolving and it has been proposed that early inhibition of the osteocyte Wnt pathway with an increase in the expression of sclerostin and other inhibitors of the Wnt/β catenin signaling pathway may be the initial stage of renal osteodystrophy and may explain observations of a relatively high and increasing prevalence of adynamic bone disease [101, 171–173]. It has even been hypothesized that in early CKD stages, low bone turnover prevails, with adynamic bone disease being the predominant form [39, 97]. With the progression of CKD to more advanced stages and increasing circulating levels of PTH, the steadily increasing activation of the PTH1R eventually overcomes the skeletal resistance to PTH and osteitis fibrosa ensues, if left untreated [12, 39]. Whether FGF23 and α-klotho play a direct role in this postulated transition from low- to high-turnover bone disease or participate only indirectly via regulating PTH secretion remains to be seen [39], but osteocyte dysfunction has been shown to be altered early in the course of CKD [39]. Of note, the use of an anti-sclerostin antibody in a CKD rat model of progressive renal osteodystrophy was shown to increase trabecular bone volume/total volume and trabecular mineralization surface in animals with low, but not high, PTH [174]. Similarly, bone properties (bone volume, cortical geometry, and biomechanical properties) improved only when PTH levels were low [174]. Whether high sclerostin levels are the cause or the consequence of PTH hyporesponsiveness in CKD remains to be clarified [166].

It also has to be taken into account that other factors such as racial and sex differences [175–177], the higher age and increased prevalence of diabetes among the CKD population, and overzealous PTH control (e.g., normalization of PTH in non-dialysis CKD patients) may influence the evaluation of PTH hyporesponsiveness [144].

Clinical Implications of Skeletal Resistance to the Action of PTH

Skeletal resistance to PTH was initially suggested as a mechanism of PTH hypersecretion in CKD. Interest in this background abnormality has been resuscitated by the effective, potentially excessive suppression of PTH by different therapies (i.e., Ca-based P binders, vitamin D, calcimimetics) and the increasing prevalence of adynamic bone disease and its associated risks (including vascular calcification and fractures) [9, 27, 60, 97, 170, 178]. As mentioned previously, skeletal resistance to PTH is currently recognized as "hyporesponsiveness" to PTH or "relative hypoparathyroidism" in terms of its relation to bone turnover [27, 39, 60, 97]. London et al., analyzing the presence of a bone–vascular axis and/or bone–vascular cross-talk [179], had already shown an inverse association between vascular calcification and lower serum PTH, low osteoclast numbers and smaller osteoblastic surfaces, and smaller or absent double tetracycline labeling surfaces, although also with high percentages of aluminum-stained surfaces [180]. In a recent cross-sectional study, these authors also found peripheral artery disease to be associated with significant reductions in the skeletal anabolic response to PTH, as demonstrated by weaker correlation coefficients (slopes) between serum PTH and double-labelled surfaces or osteoblast surfaces in patients with peripheral artery disease [181].

Additional evidence that PTH hyporesponsiveness is an important factor in the development of SHPT and/or adynamic bone disease derives from clinical studies demonstrating that a high level of circulating PTH is necessary to maintain normal bone remodeling [182–184]. Consequently, for instance in dialysis patients, current guidelines [4, 185] suggest that treatment should be modified to keep PTH levels higher than twice the upper limit of normal (better in conjunction with evaluation of bone-specific alkaline phosphatase) to avoid a low bone turnover. Also, "predialysis patients" with CKD need higher levels of PTH to maintain a normal osteoblastic surface [183], a fact that suggests that maintenance dialysis may enhance the skeletal response to PTH. However, reversibility by dialysis is not a uniform observation [52]. Finally, the presence of this multifactorial complex hyporesponsiveness to PTH may also explain the absence of clear associations between circulating PTH levels and outcomes in CKD patients (usually U-, J-, or inverted J-shaped, and overall rather weak) as opposed to the linear associations observed in primary hyperparathyroidism [27].

Conclusion

According to the previously described experimental observations demonstrating the presence of a decreased calcemic response using a PTH infusion, either with extracts in CKD patients or with synthetic PTH in different experimental models, hyporesponsiveness to PTH is just as much an integral component of CKD-MBD as are elevated circulating PTH levels [27]. Clear differences in the calcemic response to PTH among CKD and normal subjects or animals cannot just be explained by the presence of distinct inactive or antagonistic PTH fragments, since all individuals and experimental animals received the same PTH compound (usually from the same batch) at a constant rate [67, 72]. Phosphate retention, calcitriol deficiency, sclerostin, and other uremic factors may play a role by desensitizing and/or down-regulating the PTHR or downstream signaling.

Although skeletal resistance to PTH was initially suggested as a mechanism of PTH hypersecretion in CKD, "hyporesponsiveness" to PTH has also been associated with the increasing prevalence of low-turnover bone disease, which is explained by, among other factors, an increasing number of elderly and diabetic patients with CKD and treatment overshooting. Therefore, hyporesponsiveness to PTH should be taken into account when treating SHPT in CKD patients and it is important to avoid the normalization of PTH levels in these patients [139, 185]; on the other hand, progressively increasing PTH levels may indicate a change from an adaptive to a maladaptive clinical situation that requires therapeutic decisions (See Fig. 2).

Defining an optimal PTH target may be challenging but accomplishable at the population level, but it may be very difficult at the individual patient level [27]. Whether it is best to wait for onset of severe SHPT before starting antiparathyroid treatment, as suggested by the recent KDIGO guidelines [4], or to avoid complete normalization of PTH levels, as suggested by others [139], remains to be determined. Probably one single PTH recommendation does not fit all CKD patients, and nephrologists will be drawn towards a more personalized and individual management by the need to take into account other factors such as age, diabetic status, presence of metabolic syndrome, fracture risk, vascular calcification, and other biochemical markers, as well as recently identified factors that require further investigation (uremic toxins, FGF23/klotho, Wnt/β-catenin, type 2 activin A receptor pathways, etc.). Interestingly, recent evidence has indicated that osteocytes are crucial cellular targets of PTH, and the concept of "osteocytic osteolysis" has been proposed as a mechanism through which PTH rapidly increases blood calcium levels [186]. One attractive mechanism through which PTH signaling in osteocytes influences skeletal remodeling is by coordinated transcriptional regulation of paracrine mediators, including SOST [myocyte enhancer factors (MEF2)] and receptor activator of NF-κB ligand (RANKL) [186]. Beyond SOST and RANKL, PTH/PTHrP signaling in osteocytes may directly influence the way osteocytes remodel their perilacunar environment to influence bone homeostasis in a cell-autonomous manner [186].

In the meantime, despite its limitations [187], no other biomarker or therapeutic strategy has been proven to be superior to PTH, and efforts seem mandatory to improve diagnosis. More frequent monitoring, enabling PTH trends to be captured, seems the appropriate way to proceed [27] until better new molecular targets and treatments become available that demonstrate proven efficacy in clinical practice [137, 188].

Finally, resistance to the biological action of several other hormones, such as insulin, calcitriol, growth hormone, and FGF23, is also a well-known feature of CKD [189–192], as is decreased expression of several other receptors (i.e. VDR, CaSR, FGFR/klotho) [15, 72, 193–201]. As a matter of fact, uremia may thus be considered a disease which extensively affects different types of receptor (uremia as a "receptor disease") [137]. Additional studies at cellular and molecular levels are needed to establish preventive and therapeutic modalities which may be of value beyond their significance for hyporesponsiveness to PTH.

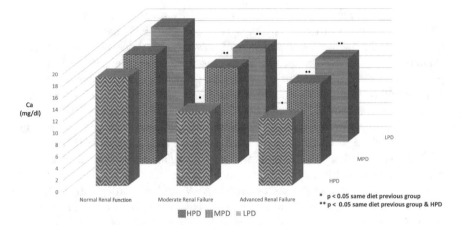

Fig. 1 Calcemic response after a 48 h PTH infusion in rats, according to different degrees of renal function (normal, moderate and advanced renal failure) and dietary phosphate (HPD: high phosphorus diet; MPD: moderate phosphorus diet; LPD: low phosphorus diet). During the PTH infusion, rats received a calcium-free-low phosphorus diet. The magnitude of the calcemic response to PTH inversely depends on the degree of renal failure and the content of phosphorus in the diet. The term "calcemic response" to PTH, "skeletal response" to PTH or "end-organ resistance" to PTH evolved to "hyporesponsiveness" to PTH (see text) Adapted from Ref. [68]

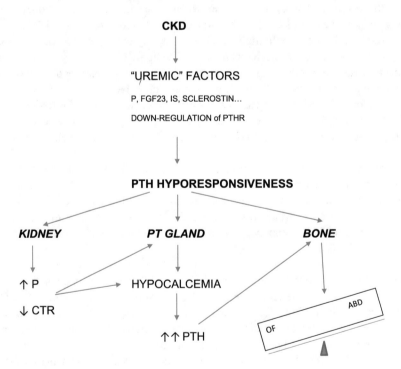

Fig. 2 Causes and consequences of parathyroid hormone (PTH) hyporesponsiveness in chronic kidney disease (CKD). P = Phosphate; FGF-23 = Fibroblast Growth Factor 23; IS = indoxyl-sulfate; PTHR = PTH receptor; PT = parathyroid; CTR = calcitriol; OF = Osteitis fibrosa; ABD = Adynamic bone disease

Table 1 Factors associated with skeletal resistance to PTH action (hyporesponsiveness to PTH)

Decreased levels of calcitriol
Phosphate retention and hyperphosphatemia
Down-regulation of PTH receptors
Uremia
PTH abnormal metabolism and PTH fragments
FGF23/klotho
Calcitonin
Osteoprotegerin
Wnt antagonists: sclerostin…
RANKL
Other: race, sex, aging, diabetes

References

1. Martínez-Castelao A, Górriz JL, Segura-de la Morena J, et al. Consensus document for the detection and management of chronic kidney disease. Nefrologia. 2014;34:243–62.
2. Covic A, Vervloet M, Massy ZA, et al. Bone and mineral disorders in chronic kidney disease: implications for cardiovascular health and ageing in the general population. Lancet Diabetes Endocrinol. 2018;6:319–31.
3. Moe SM, Drueke T, Lameire N, Eknoyan G. Chronic kidney disease-mineral bone disorder: a new paradigm. Adv Chronic Kidney Dis. 2007;14:3–12.
4. Kidney Disease: Improving Global Outcomes (KDIGO) CKD-MBD Update Work Group. KDIGO 2017 clinical practice guideline update for the diagnosis, evaluation, prevention, and treatment of chronic kidney disease-mineral and bone disorder (CKD-MBD). Kidney Int Suppl. 2017;7:1–59.
5. Cozzolino M, Urena-Torres P, Vervloet MG, Brandenburg V, Bover J, Goldsmith D, Larsson TE, Massy ZA, Mazzaferro S. Is chronic kidney disease-mineral bone disorder (CKD-MBD) really a syndrome? Nephrol Dial Transpl. 2014;29:1815–20.
6. Vervloet MG, Massy ZA, Brandenburg VM, Mazzaferro S, Cozzolino M, Ureña-Torres P, Bover J, Goldsmith D. Bone: a new endocrine organ at the heart of chronic kidney disease and mineral and bone disorders. Lancet Diabetes Endocrinol. 2014;2:427–36.
7. Rodriguez M, Salmeron MD, Martin-Malo A, Barbieri C, Mari F, Molina RI, Costa P, Aljama P. A new data analysis system to quantify associations between biochemical parameters of chronic kidney disease-mineral bone disease. PLoS ONE. 2016;11:e0146801.
8. Behets GJ, Spasovski G, Sterling LR, Goodman WG, Spiegel DM, De Broe ME, D'Haese PC. Bone histomorphometry before and after long-term treatment with cinacalcet in dialysis patients with secondary hyperparathyroidism. Kidney Int. 2015;87:846–56.
9. Noordzij M, Cranenburg EM, Engelsman LF, et al. Progression of aortic calcification is associated with disorders of mineral metabolism and mortality in chronic dialysis patients. Nephrol Dial Transpl. 2011;26:1662–9.
10. Massry SG. Is parathyroid hormone a uremic toxin? Nephron. 1977;19:125–30.
11. Rodriguez M, Lorenzo V. Parathyroid hormone, a uremic toxin. Semin Dial. 2009;22:363–8.
12. Ureña-Torres PA, Vervloet M, Mazzaferro S, Oury F, Brandenburg V, Bover J et al. Novel insights into parathyroid hormone: report of The Parathyroid Day in chronic kidney disease. Clin Kidney J. 2018. https://doi.org/10.1093/ckj/sfy061 (Epub ahead online: https://academic.oup.com/ckj/advance-article/doi/10.1093/ckj/sfy061/5056879).
13. Slatopolsky E, Martin K, Hruska K. Parathyroid hormone metabolism and its potential as a uremic toxin. Am J Physiol Physiol. 1980;239:F1–12.
14. Morii H, Nishizawa Y, Smogorzewski M, Inaba M, Massry SG. New actions of parathyroid hormone. Introduction. Miner Electrolyte Metab. 1995;21:7–8.

15. Llach F, Bover J. Renal Osteodystrophies. In: Brenner BM, editor. The kidney, 6th ed. Philadelphia: W.B. Saunders Company;2000. p. 2103–2186.
16. Vaidya A, Brown JM, Williams JS. The renin–angiotensin–aldosterone system and calcium-regulatory hormones. J Hum Hypertens. 2015;29:515–21.
17. Kir S, Komaba H, Garcia AP, Economopoulos KP, Liu W, Lanske B, Hodin RA, Spiegelman BM. PTH/PTHrP receptor mediates cachexia in models of kidney failure and cancer. Cell Metab. 2016;23:315–23.
18. McMahon DJ, Carrelli A, Palmeri N, Zhang C, DiTullio M, Silverberg SJ, Walker MD. Effect of parathyroidectomy upon left ventricular mass in primary hyperparathyroidism: a meta-analysis. J Clin Endocrinol Metab. 2015;100:4399–407.
19. Seiler-Mussler S, Limbach AS, Emrich IE, Pickering JW, Roth HJ, Fliser D, Heine GH. Association of nonoxidized parathyroid hormone with cardiovascular and kidney disease outcomes in chronic kidney disease. Clin J Am Soc Nephrol. 2018;13:569–76.
20. Floege J, Kim J, Ireland E, et al. Serum iPTH, calcium and phosphate, and the risk of mortality in a European haemodialysis population. Nephrol Dial Transpl. 2011;26:1948–55.
21. Young EW, Akiba T, Albert JM, McCarthy JT, Kerr PG, Mendelssohn DC, Jadoul M. Magnitude and impact of abnormal mineral metabolism in hemodialysis patients in the Dialysis Outcomes and Practice Patterns Study (DOPPS). Am J Kidney Dis. 2004;44:34–8.
22. Ureña Torres PA, De Broe M. Calcium-sensing receptor, calcimimetics, and cardiovascular calcifications in chronic kidney disease. Kidney Int. 2012;82:19–25.
23. Wheeler DC, London GM, Parfrey PS, Block GA, Correa-Rotter R, Dehmel B, Drücke TB, Floege J, Kubo Y, Mahaffey KW, Goodman WG, Moe SM, Trotman ML, Abdalla S, Chertow GM, Herzog CA. Effects of cinacalcet on atherosclerotic and nonatherosclerotic cardiovascular events in patients receiving hemodialysis: the EValuation Of Cinacalcet HCl Therapy to Lower CardioVascular Events (EVOLVE) trial. J Am Heart Assoc. 2012;4(1):e000570.
24. Joy MS, Karagiannis PC, Peyerl FW. Outcomes of secondary hyperparathyroidism in chronic kidney disease and the direct costs of treatment. J Manag Care Pharm. 2007;13:397–411.
25. Fernández-Martín JL, Martínez-Camblor P, Dionisi MP, Floege J, Ketteler M, London G, Locatelli F, Gorriz JL, Rutkowski B, Ferreira A, Bos WJ, Covic A, Rodríguez-García M, Sánchez JE, Rodríguez-Puyol D, Cannata-Andia JB, COSMOS group. Improvement of mineral and bone metabolism markers is associated with better survival in haemodialysis patients: the COSMOS study. Nephrol Dial Transplant. 2015;30(9):1542–51.
26. Kurz P, Monier-Faugere MC, Bognar B, Werner E, Roth P, Vlachojannis J, Malluche HH. Evidence for abnormal calcium homeostasis in patients with adynamic bone disease. Kidney Int. 1994;46:855–61.
27. Evenepoel P, Bover J, Ureña Torres P. Parathyroid hormone metabolism and signaling in health and chronic kidney disease. Kidney Int. 2016;90:1184–90.
28. Kidney Disease: Improving Global Outcomes (KDIGO) CKD-MBD Update Work Group. KDIGO clinical practice guideline for the diagnosis, evaluation, prevention, and treatment of Chronic Kidney Disease-Mineral and Bone Disorder (CKD-MBD). Kidney Int Suppl. 2009;76:S1–130.
29. Kazama JJ, Iwasaki Y, Fukagawa M. Uremic osteoporosis. Kidney Int Suppl. 2013;3:446–50.
30. Kazama JJ, Matsuo K, Iwasaki Y, Fukagawa M. Chronic kidney disease and bone metabolism. J Bone Miner Metab. 2015;33:245–52.
31. Pilz S, Tomaschitz A, Drechsler C, Ritz E, Boehm BO, Grammer TB, Marz W. Parathyroid hormone level is associated with mortality and cardiovascular events in patients undergoing coronary angiography. Eur Heart J. 2010;31:1591–8.
32. London G. Cardiovascular disease in end-stage renal failure: role of calcium-phosphate disturbances and hyperparathyroidism. J Nephrol. 2002;15:209–10.
33. London GM, De Vernejoul MC, Fabiani F, Marchais SJ, Guerin AP, Metivier F, London AM, Llach F. Secondary hyperparathyroidism and cardiac hypertrophy in hemodialysis patients. Kidney Int. 1987;32:900–7.

34. Slatopolsky E, Caglar S, Pennell JP, Taggart DD, Canterbury JM, Reiss E, Bricker NS. On the pathogenesis of hyperparathyroidism in chronic experimental renal insufficiency in the dog. J Clin Invest. 1971;50:492–9.
35. Slatopolsky E, Bricker NS. The role of phosphorus restriction in the prevention of secondary hyperparathyroidism in chronic renal disease. Kidney Int. 1973;4:141–5.
36. Kuro-o M. Klotho, phosphate and FGF-23 in ageing and disturbed mineral metabolism. Nat Rev Nephrol. 2013;9:650–60.
37. Kuro-o M, Moe OW. FGF23-αKlotho as a paradigm for a kidney-bone network. Bone. 2017;100:4–18.
38. Wolf M. Forging forward with 10 burning questions on FGF23 in kidney disease. J Am Soc Nephrol. 2010;21:1427–35.
39. Drüeke TB, Massy ZA. Changing bone patterns with progression of chronic kidney disease. Kidney Int. 2016;89:289–302.
40. Hruska KA, Sugatani T, Agapova O, Fang Y. The chronic kidney disease—mineral bone disorder (CKD-MBD): advances in pathophysiology. Bone. 2017;100:80–6.
41. Cunningham J, Locatelli F, Rodriguez M. Secondary hyperparathyroidism: pathogenesis, disease progression, and therapeutic options. Clin J Am Soc Nephrol. 2011;6:913–21.
42. Rodriguez M, Nemeth E, Martin D. The calcium-sensing receptor: a key factor in the pathogenesis of secondary hyperparathyroidism. Am J Physiol Renal Physiol. 2005;288:F253–64.
43. Tominaga Y, Takagi H. Molecular genetics of hyperparathyroid disease. Curr Opin Nephrol Hypertens. 1996;5:336–41.
44. Almaden Y, Canalejo A, Hernandez A, Ballesteros E, Garcia-Navarro S, Torres A, Rodriguez M, Rodriguez M. Direct effect of phosphorus on PTH secretion from whole rat parathyroid glands in vitro. J Bone Miner Res. 1996;11:970–6.
45. Almaden Y, Hernandez A, Torregrosa V, Canalejo A, Sabate L, Fernandez Cruz L, Campistol JM, Torres A, Rodriguez M. High phosphate level directly stimulates parathyroid hormone secretion and synthesis by human parathyroid tissue in vitro. J Am Soc Nephrol. 1998;9:1845–52.
46. Slatopolsky E, Finch J, Denda M, Ritter C, Zhong M, Dusso A, MacDonald PN, Brown AJ. Phosphorus restriction prevents parathyroid gland growth. High phosphorus directly stimulates PTH secretion in vitro. J Clin Invest. 1996;97:2534–40.
47. Rodriguez-Ortiz ME, Lopez I, Muñoz-Castañeda JR, et al. Calcium deficiency reduces circulating levels of FGF23. J Am Soc Nephrol. 2012;23:1190–7.
48. Mace ML, Gravesen E, Nordholm A, Olgaard K, Lewin E. Fibroblast Growth Factor (FGF) 23 regulates the plasma levels of parathyroid hormone in vivo through the FGF receptor in normocalcemia, but not in hypocalcemia. Calcif Tissue Int. 2018;102:85–92.
49. Evanson JM. The response to the infusion of parathyroid extract in hypocalcaemic states. Clin Sci. 1966;31:63–75.
50. Kruse K, Kracht U, Wohlfart K, Kruse U. Biochemical markers of bone turnover, intact serum parathyroid hormone and renal calcium excretion in patients with pseudohypoparathyroidism and hypoparathyroidism before and during vitamin D treatment. Eur J Pediatr. 1989;148:535–9.
51. Massry SG, Stein R, Garty J, Arieff AI, Coburn JW, Norman AW, Friedler RM. Skeletal resistance to the calcemic action of parathyroid hormone in uremia: role of 1,25 (OH)2 D3. Kidney Int. 1976;9:467–74.
52. Massry SG, Coburn JW, Lee DB, Jowsey J, Kleeman CR. Skeletal resistance to parathyroid hormone in renal failure. Studies in 105 human subjects. Ann Intern Med. 1973;78:357–64.
53. Llach F, Massry SG, Singer FR, Kurokawa K, Kaye JH, Coburn JW. Skeletal resistance to endogenous parathyroid hormone in patients with early renal failure. A possible cause for secondary hyperparathyroidism. J Clin Endocrinol Metab. 1975;41:339–45.
54. Wilson L, Felsenfeld A, Drezner MK, Llach F. Altered divalent ion metabolism in early renal failure: role of 1,25(OH)2D. Kidney Int. 1985;27:565–73.
55. Albright F, Drake TG, Sulkowitch HW. Renal osteitis fibrosa cystica. Bull Johns Hopkins Hosp. 1937;60:377–99.

56. Bricker NS, Slatopolsky E, Reiss E, Avioli LV. Calcium, phosphorus, and bone in renal disease and transplantation. Arch Intern Med. 1969;123:543–53.
57. Slatopolsky E, Caglar S, Gradowska L, Canterbury J, Reiss E, Bricker NS. On the prevention of secondary hyperparathyroidism in experimental chronic renal disease using proportional reduction of dietary phosphorus intake. Kidney Int. 1972;2:147–51.
58. Deykin D, Balko C, Bricker NS. On the pathogenesis of the uremic state. N Engl J Med. 1972;286:1093–9.
59. Llach F. Secondary hyperparathyroidism in renal failure: the trade-off hypothesis revisited. Am J Kidney Dis. 1995;25:663–79.
60. Fukagawa M, Kazama JJ, Shigematsu T. Skeletal resistance to PTH as a basic abnormality underlying uremic bone diseases. Am J Kidney Dis. 2001;38:S152–5.
61. Levin A, Bakris GL, Molitch M, Smulders M, Tian J, Williams LA, Andress DL. Prevalence of abnormal serum vitamin D, PTH, calcium, and phosphorus in patients with chronic kidney disease: results of the study to evaluate early kidney disease. Kidney Int. 2007;71:31–8.
62. Somerville PJ, Kaye M. Resistance to parathyroid hormone in renal failure: role of vitamin D metabolites. Kidney Int. 1978;14:245–54.
63. Rodriguez M, Felsenfeld AJ, Llach F. Calcemic response to parathyroid hormone in renal failure: role of calcitriol and the effect of parathyroidectomy. Kidney Int. 1991;40:1063–8.
64. Massry SG, Tuma S, Dua S, Goldstein DA. Reversal of skeletal resistance to parathyroid hormone in uremia by vitamin D metabolites: evidence for the requirement of 1,25(OH)2D3 and 24,25(OH)2D3. J Lab Clin Med. 1979;94:152–7.
65. Galceran T, Martin KJ, Morrissey JJ, Slatopolsky E. Role of 1,25-dihydroxyvitamin D on the skeletal resistance to parathyroid hormone. Kidney Int. 1987;32:801–7.
66. Somerville PJ, Kaye M. Evidence that resistance to the calcemic action of parathyroid hormone in rats with acute uremia is caused by phosphate retention. Kidney Int. 1979;16:552–60.
67. Bover J, Rodriguez M, Trinidad P, Jara A, Martinez ME, Machado L, Llach F, Felsenfeld AJ. Factors in the development of secondary hyperparathyroidism during graded renal failure in the rat. Kidney Int. 1994;45:953–61.
68. Bover J, Jara A, Trinidad P, Rodriguez M, Felsenfeld AJ. Dynamics of skeletal resistance to parathyroid hormone in the rat: effect of renal failure and dietary phosphorus. Bone. 1999;25:279–85.
69. Llach F, Massry SG. On the mechanism of secondary hyperparathyroidism in moderate renal insufficiency. J Clin Endocrinol Metab. 1985;61:601–6.
70. Yates AJ, Oreffo RO, Mayor K, Mundy GR. Inhibition of bone resorption by inorganic phosphate is mediated by both reduced osteoclast formation and decreased activity of mature osteoclasts. J Bone Miner Res. 1991;6:473–8.
71. Geng Y, Mosyak L, Kurinov I, et al. Structural mechanism of ligand activation in human calcium-sensing receptor. eLife. 2016;5;pii:e13662.
72. Bover J, Jara A, Trinidad P, Rodriguez M, Martin-Malo A, Felsenfeld AJ. The calcemic response to PTH in the rat: effect of elevated PTH levels and uremia. Kidney Int. 1994;46:310–7.
73. Fujimori A, Miyauchi A, Hruska KA, Martin KJ, Avioli LV, Civitelli R. Desensitization of calcium messenger system in parathyroid hormone-stimulated opossum kidney cells. Am J Physiol. 1993;264:E918–24.
74. Olgaard K, Arbelaez M, Schwartz J, Klahr S, Slatopolsky E. Abnormal skeletal response to parathyroid hormone in dogs with chronic uremia. Calcif Tissue Int. 1982;34:403–7.
75. Olgaard K, Schwartz J, Finco D, Arbelaez M, Korkor A, Martin K, Klahr S, Slatopolsky E. Extraction of parathyroid hormone and release of adenosine 3',5'-monophosphate by isolated perfused bones obtained from dogs with acute uremia. Endocrinology. 1982;111:1678–82.
76. Roth J, Grunfeld C. Endocrine systems: mechanisms of disease, target cells, and receptors. In: RH Williams, editor. Textbook of endocrinology, 6th ed. Philadelphia: W.B. Saunders Comp., Williams & Wilkins;1981. p. 41–3.

77. Drüeke TB. Abnormal skeletal response to parathyroid hormone and the expression of its receptor in chronic uremia. Pediatr Nephrol. 1996;10:348–50.
78. Jüppner H, Abou-Samra AB, Freeman M, Kong XF, Schipani E, Richards J, Kolakowski LF, Hock J, Potts JT, Kronenberg HM. A G protein-linked receptor for parathyroid hormone and parathyroid hormone-related peptide. Science. 1991;254:1024–6.
79. Abou-Samra AB, Jüppner H, Force T, Freeman MW, Kong XF, Schipani E, Urena P, Richards J, Bonventre JV, Potts JT. Expression cloning of a common receptor for parathyroid hormone and parathyroid hormone-related peptide from rat osteoblast-like cells: a single receptor stimulates intracellular accumulation of both cAMP and inositol trisphosphates and increases intracellular free calcium. Proc Natl Acad Sci U S A. 1992;89:2732–6.
80. Ureña P, Kong XF, Abou-Samra AB, Jüppner H, Kronenberg HM, Potts JT, Segre GV. Parathyroid hormone (PTH)/PTH-related peptide receptor messenger ribonucleic acids are widely distributed in rat tissues. Endocrinology. 1993;133:617–23.
81. Iwasaki-Ishizuka Y, Yamato H, Nii-Kono T, Kurokawa K, Fukagawa M. Downregulation of parathyroid hormone receptor gene expression and osteoblastic dysfunction associated with skeletal resistance to parathyroid hormone in a rat model of renal failure with low turnover bone. Nephrol Dial Transplant. 2005;20:1904–11.
82. Ureña P, Kubrusly M, Mannstadt M, Hruby M, Trinh MM, Silve C, Lacour B, Abou-Samra AB, Segre GV, Drüeke T. The renal PTH/PTHrP receptor is down-regulated in rats with chronic renal failure. Kidney Int. 1994;45:605–11.
83. Tian J, Smogorzewski M, Kedes L, Massry SG. PTH-PTHrP receptor mRNA is downregulated in chronic renal failure. Am J Nephrol. 1994;14:41–6.
84. Ureña P, Ferreira A, Morieux C, Drüeke T, de Vernejoul MC. PTH/PTHrP receptor mRNA is down-regulated in epiphyseal cartilage growth plate of uraemic rats. Nephrol Dial Transpl. 1996;11:2008–16.
85. Picton ML, Moore PR, Mawer EB, Houghton D, Freemont AJ, Hutchison AJ, Gokal R, Hoyland JA. Down-regulation of human osteoblast PTH/PTHrP receptor mRNA in end-stage renal failure. Kidney Int. 2000;58:1440–9.
86. Pereira RC, Delany AM, Khouzam NM, Bowen RE, Freymiller EG, Salusky IB, Wesseling-Perry K. Primary osteoblast-like cells from patients with end-stage kidney disease reflect gene expression, proliferation, and mineralization characteristics ex vivo. Kidney Int. 2015;87:593–601.
87. Ureña P, Mannstadt M, Hruby M, Ferreira A, Schmitt F, Silve C, Ardaillou R, Lacour B, Abou-Samra AB, Segre GV. Parathyroidectomy does not prevent the renal PTH/PTHrP receptor down-regulation in uremic rats. Kidney Int. 1995;47:1797–805.
88. Sanchez C, Salusky I, Willsey P et al. Calcitriol upregulates PTH/PTHrP receptor mRNA in rat growth plate cartilage. J Am Soc Nephrol. 1995;6:970 (Abstract).
89. Gonzalez EA MK. Calcitriol decreases PTH/PTHrp receptor gene expression in UMR 106-01 cells. J Am Soc Nephrol. 1994);5:880 (Abstract).
90. Zoccali C, Mallamaci F LD et al. Autoregulation of PTH secretion. J Am Soc Nephrol. 1994;5:892 (Abstract).
91. Suarez-Bregua P, Cal L, Cañestro C, Rotllant J. PTH reloaded: a new evolutionary perspective. Front Physiol. 2017;8:776.
92. Berdud I, Martin-Malo A, Almaden Y, Tallon S, Concepcion MT, Torres A, Felsenfeld A, Aljama P, Rodriguez M. Abnormal calcaemic response to PTH in the uraemic rat without secondary hyperparathyroidism. Nephrol Dial Transpl. 1996;11:1292–8.
93. Wills MR, Jenkins MV. The effect of uraemic metabolites on parathyroid extract-induced bone resorption in vitro. Clin Chim Acta. 1976;73:121–5.
94. Andress DL, Howard GA, Birnbaum RS. Identification of a low molecular weight inhibitor of osteoblast mitogenesis in uremic plasma. Kidney Int. 1991;39:942–5.
95. Disthabanchong S, Hassan H, McConkey CL, Martin KJ, Gonzalez EA. Regulation of PTH1 receptor expression by uremic ultrafiltrate in UMR 106–01 osteoblast-like cells. Kidney Int. 2004;65:897–903.

96. Nii-Kono T, Iwasaki Y, Uchida M, Fujieda A, Hosokawa A, Motojima M, Yamato H, Kurokawa K, Fukagawa M. Indoxyl sulfate induces skeletal resistance to parathyroid hormone in cultured osteoblastic cells. Kidney Int. 2007;71:738–43.

97. Massy Z, Drueke T. Adynamic bone disease is a predominant bone pattern in early stages of chronic kidney disease. J Nephrol. 2017;30:629–34.

98. Sage AP, Lu J, Atti E, Tetradis S, Ascenzi M-G, Adams DJ, Demer LL, Tintut Y. Hyperlipidemia induces resistance to PTH bone anabolism in mice via oxidized lipids. J Bone Miner Res. 2011;26:1197–206.

99. Mozar A, Louvet L, Godin C, Mentaverri R, Brazier M, Kamel S, Massy ZA. Indoxyl sulphate inhibits osteoclast differentiation and function. Nephrol Dial Transpl. 2012;27:2176–81.

100. Iwasaki Y, Yamato H, Nii-Kono T, Fujieda A, Uchida M, Hosokawa A, Motojima M, Fukagawa M. Administration of oral charcoal adsorbent (AST-120) suppresses low-turnover bone progression in uraemic rats. Nephrol Dial Transpl. 2006;21:2768–74.

101. Barreto FC, Barreto DV, Canziani MEF, Tomiyama C, Higa A, Mozar A, Glorieux G, Vanholder R, Massy Z, Carvalho AB. Association between indoxyl sulfate and bone histomorphometry in pre-dialysis chronic kidney disease patients. J Bras Nefrol. 2014;36:289–96.

102. Hsu CH, Patel S. Uremic plasma contains factors inhibiting 1 alpha-hydroxylase activity. J Am Soc Nephrol. 1992;3:947–52.

103. Patel SR, Ke HQ, Vanholder R, Koenig RJ, Hsu CH. Inhibition of calcitriol receptor binding to vitamin D response elements by uremic toxins. J Clin Invest. 1995;96:50–9.

104. Habener JF, Potts JT. Biosynthesis of parathyroid hormone. N Engl J Med. 1978;299:635–44.

105. Kakuta T, Sawada K. New developments in CKD-MBD. Cell biology of parathyroid in CKD. Clin Calcium. 2014;24:1801–8.

106. Basile C, Lomonte C. The function of the parathyroid oxyphil cells in uremia: still a mystery? Kidney Int. 2017;92:1046–8.

107. Ritter C, Miller B, Coyne DW, Gupta D, Zheng S, Brown AJ, Slatopolsky E. Paricalcitol and cinacalcet have disparate actions on parathyroid oxyphil cell content in patients with chronic kidney disease. Kidney Int. 2017;92:1217–22.

108. Kitamura N, Shigeno C, Shiomi K, et al. Episodic fluctuation in serum intact parathyroid hormone concentration in men. J Clin Endocrinol Metab. 1990;70:252–63.

109. Tam CS, Heersche JNM, Murray TM, Parsons JA. Parathyroid hormone stimulates the bone apposition rate independently of its resorptive action: differential effects of intermittent and continuous administration. Endocrinology. 1982;110:506–12.

110. Hock JM, Gera I. Effects of continuous and intermittent administration and inhibition of resorption on the anabolic response of bone to parathyroid hormone. J Bone Miner Res. 1992;7:65–72.

111. de Francisco AL, Amado JA, Cotorruelo JG, González M, de Castro SS, Canga E, de Bonis E, Ruiz JC, Arias M, Gonzalez-Macías J. Pulsatile-secretion of parathyroid hormone in patients with chronic renal failure. Clin Nephrol. 1993;39:224–8.

112. Hocher B, Zeng S. Clear the fog around parathyroid hormone assays: what do iPTH assays really measure? Clin J Am Soc Nephrol. 2018;13:524–6.

113. Tregear GW, Van Rietschoten J, Greene E, Keutmann HT, Niall HD, Reit B, Parsons JA, Potts JT. Bovine parathyroid hormone: minimum chain length of synthetic peptide required for biological activity. Endocrinology. 1973;93:1349–53.

114. Lim SK, Gardella TJ, Baba H, Nussbaum SR, Kronenberg HM. The carboxy-terminus of parathyroid hormone is essential for hormone processing and secretion. Endocrinology. 1992;131:2325–30.

115. Maye GP, Keaton JA, Hurst JG, Habener JF. Effects of plasma calcium concentration on the relative proportion of hormone and carboxyl fragments in parathyroid venous blood. Endocrinology. 1979;104:1778–84.

116. Santamaria R, Almaden Y, Felsenfeld A, Martin-Malo A, Gao P, Cantor T, Aljama P, Rodriguez M. Dynamics of PTH secretion in hemodialysis patients as determined by the intact and whole PTH assays. Kidney Int. 2003;64:1867–73.

117. Brossard JH, Whittom S, Lepage R, D'Amour P. Carboxyl-terminal fragments of parathyroid hormone are not secreted preferentially in primary hyperparathyroidism as they are in other hypercalcemic conditions. J Clin Endocrinol Metab. 1993;77:413–9.

118. el-Hajj Fuleihan G, Chen CJ, Rivkees SA, Marynick SP, Stock J, Pallotta JA, Brown EM. Calcium-dependent release of N-terminal fragments and intact immunoreactive parathyroid hormone by human pathological parathyroid tissue in vitro. J Clin Endocrinol Metab. 1989;69:860–7.

119. Catherwood BD, Friedler RM, Singer FR. Sites of clearance of endogenous parathyroid hormone in the vitamin D-deficient dog. Endocrinology. 1976;98:228–36.

120. Martin K, Hruska K, Greenwalt A, Klahr S, Slatopolsky E. Selective uptake of intact parathyroid hormone by the liver: differences between hepatic and renal uptake. J Clin Invest. 1976;58:781–8.

121. Martin KJ, Hruska KA, Lewis J, Anderson C, Slatopolsky E. The renal handling of parathyroid hormone. Role of peritubular uptake and glomerular filtration. J Clin Invest. 1977;60:808–14.

122. Zull JE, Chuang J. Characterization of parathyroid hormone fragments produced by cathepsin D. J Biol Chem. 1985;260:1608–13.

123. Freitag J, Martin KJ, Hruska KA, Anderson C, Conrades M, Ladenson J, Klahr S, Slatopolsky E. Impaired parathyroid hormone metabolism in patients with chronic renal failure. N Engl J Med. 1978;298:29–32.

124. Brossard JH, Cloutier M, Roy L, Lepage R, Gascon-Barré M, D'Amour P. Accumulation of a non-(1-84) molecular form of parathyroid hormone (PTH) detected by intact PTH assay in renal failure: importance in the interpretation of PTH values. J Clin Endocrinol Metab. 1996;81:3923–9.

125. Lepage R, Roy L, Brossard JH, Rousseau L, Dorais C, Lazure C, D'Amour P. A non-(1-84) circulating parathyroid hormone (PTH) fragment interferes significantly with intact PTH commercial assay measurements in uremic samples. Clin Chem. 1998;44:805–9.

126. Cavalier E, Delanaye P, Vranken L, Bekaert AC, Carlisi A, Chapelle JP, Souberbielle JC. Interpretation of serum PTH concentrations with different kits in dialysis patients according to the KDIGO guidelines: importance of the reference (normal) values. Nephrol Dial Transpl. 2012;27:1950–6.

127. Souberbielle JC, Friedlander G, Cormier C. Practical considerations in PTH testing. Clin Chim Acta. 2006;366:81–9.

128. Souberbielle JCP, Roth H, Fouque DP. Parathyroid hormone measurement in CKD. Kidney Int. 2010;77:93–100.

129. Souberbielle JC, Boutten A, Carlier MC, et al. Inter-method variability in PTH measurement: implication for the care of CKD patients. Kidney Int. 2006;70:345–50.

130. Slatopolsky E, Finch J, Clay P, Martin D, Sicard G, Singer G, Gao P, Cantor T, Dusso A. A novel mechanism for skeletal resistance in uremia. Kidney Int. 2000;58:753–61.

131. Malluche HH, Mawad H, Trueba D, Monier-Faugere MC. Parathyroid hormone assays–evolution and revolutions in the care of dialysis patients. Clin Nephrol. 2003;59:313–8.

132. González-Casaus ML, González-Parra E, Sánchez-González C, Albalate M, de la Piedra-Gordo C, Fernández E, Torregrosa V, Rodríguez M, Lorenzo V. A lower proportion of circulating active parathyroid hormone in peritoneal dialysis does not allow the pth inter-method adjustment proposed for haemodialysis. Nefrologia. 2014;34:330–40.

133. Hocher B, Armbruster FP, Stoeva S, Reichetzeder C, Grön HJ, Lieker I, Khadzhynov D, Slowinski T, Roth HJ. Measuring Parathyroid Hormone (PTH) in patients with oxidative stress—do we need a fourth generation parathyroid hormone assay? PLoS ONE. 2012;7:e40242.

134. Hocher B, Oberthür D, Slowinski T, et al. Modeling of oxidized PTH (oxPTH) and non-oxidized PTH (n-oxPTH) receptor binding and relationship of oxidized to non-oxidized PTH in children with chronic renal failure, adult patients on hemodialysis and kidney transplant recipients. Kidney Blood Press Res. 2013;37:240–51.
135. Tepel M, Armbruster FP, Grön HJ, Scholze A, Reichetzeder C, Roth HJ, Hocher B. Nonoxidized, biologically active parathyroid hormone determines mortality in hemodialysis patients. J Clin Endocrinol Metab. 2013;98:4744–51.
136. Souberbielle JC, Massart C, Brailly-Tabard S, Cormier C, Cavalier E, Delanaye P, Chanson P. Serum PTH reference values established by an automated third-generation assay in vitamin D-replete subjects with normal renal function: consequences of diagnosing primary hyperparathyroidism and the classification of dialysis patients. Eur J Endocrinol. 2016;174:315–23.
137. Bover J, Ureña P, Aguilar A, Mazzaferro S, Benito S, López-Báez V, Ramos A, daSilva I, Cozzolino M. Alkaline phosphatases in the complex chronic kidney disease-mineral and bone disorders. Calcif Tissue Int. 2018;103:111–24.
138. Tolouian RGA. The need for a reliable bone biomarker to better assess chronic kidney disease mineral and bone disorder. J Parathyr Dis. 2018;6:36–8.
139. Torregrosa V, Bover J, Cannata J et al. Spanish Society of Nephrology recommendations for controlling mineral and bone disorder in chronic kidney disease patients (S.E.N.-M.B.D.). Nefrologia. 2019 (submitted).
140. Divieti P, John MR, Jüppner H, Bringhurst FR. Human PTH-(7-84) inhibits bone resorption in vitro via actions independent of the type 1 PTH/PTHrP receptor. Endocrinology. 2002;143:171–6.
141. Nguyen M, He B, Karaplis A. Nuclear forms of parathyroid hormone-related peptide are translated from non-AUG start sites downstream from the initiator methionine. Endocrinology. 2001;142:694–703.
142. Murray TM, Rao LG, Divieti P, Bringhurst FR. Parathyroid hormone secretion and action: evidence for discrete receptors for the carboxyl-terminal region and related biological actions of carboxyl-terminal ligands. Endocr Rev. 2005;26:78–113.
143. Inomata N, Akiyama M, Kubota N, Jüppner H. Characterization of a novel parathyroid hormone (PTH) receptor with specificity for the carboxyl-terminal region of PTH-(1-84). Endocrinology. 1995;136:4732–40.
144. Wesseling-Perry K, Harkins GC, Wang H, Elashoff R, Gales B, Horwitz MJ, Stewart AF, Jüppner H, Salusky IB. The calcemic response to continuous parathyroid hormone (PTH) (1-34) infusion in end-stage kidney disease varies according to bone turnover: a potential role for PTH(7-84). J Clin Endocrinol Metab. 2010;95:2772–80.
145. Huan J, Olgaard K, Nielsen LB, Lewin E. Parathyroid hormone 7-84 induces hypocalcemia and inhibits the parathyroid hormone 1-84 secretory response to hypocalcemia in rats with intact parathyroid glands. J Am Soc Nephrol. 2006;17:1923–30.
146. Behar V, Pines M, Nakamoto C, et al. The human PTH2 receptor: binding and signal transduction properties of the stably expressed recombinant receptor. Endocrinology. 1996;137:2748–57.
147. Ureña P. The PTH/PTHrP receptor: biological implications. Nefrologia. 2003;23(Suppl 2):12–7.
148. Takenaka T, Inoue T, Miyazaki T, Hayashi M, Suzuki H. Xeno-klotho inhibits parathyroid hormone signaling. J Bone Miner Res. 2016;31:455–62.
149. Torres A, Rodriguez M, Felsenfeld A, Martin-Malo A, Llach F. Sigmoidal relationship between calcitonin and calcium: studies in normal, parathyroidectomized, and azotemic rats. Kidney Int. 1991;40:700–4.
150. Felsenfeld AJ, Machado L, Rodriguez M. The relationship between serum calcitonin and calcium in the hemodialysis patient. Am J Kidney Dis. 1993;21:292–9.
151. Rodriguez M, Felsenfeld AJ, Torres A, Pederson L, Llach F. Calcitonin, an important factor in the calcemic response to parathyroid hormone in the rat. Kidney Int. 1991;40:219–25.

152. Quesada JM, Rodriguez M, Calderon de la Barca JM, Alvarez-Lara A, Martín-Malo A, Mateo A, Martinez ME, Aljama P. Effect of calcitriol replacement on serum calcitonin and parathyroid hormone levels in CAPD patients. Nephrol Dial Transpl. 1995;10:70–4.
153. Arenas MD, de la Fuente V, Delgado P, Gil MT, Gutiérrez P, Ribero J, Rodríguez M, Almadén Y. Pharmacodynamics of cinacalcet over 48 hours in patients with controlled secondary hyperparathyroidism: useful data in clinical practice. J Clin Endocrinol Metab. 2013;98:1718–25.
154. Felsenfeld A, Rodriguez M, Levine B. New insights in regulation of calcium homeostasis. Curr Opin Nephrol Hypertens. 2013;22:371–6.
155. Kazama JJ. The skeletal resistance to PTH and osteoprotegerin. Clin Calcium. 2002;12:764–7.
156. Kim CS, Bae EH, Ma SK, et al. Association of Serum Osteoprotegerin Levels with bone loss in chronic kidney disease: insights from the KNOW-CKD study. PLoS ONE. 2016;11:e0166792.
157. Kazama JJ, Shigematsu T, Yano K, Tsuda E, Miura M, Iwasaki Y, Kawaguchi Y, Gejyo F, Kurokawa K, Fukagawa M. Increased circulating levels of osteoclastogenesis inhibitory factor (osteoprotegerin) in patients with chronic renal failure. Am J Kidney Dis. 2002;39:525–32.
158. Winkler DG, Sutherland MK, Geoghegan JC, et al. Osteocyte control of bone formation via sclerostin, a novel BMP antagonist. EMBO J. 2003;22:6267–76.
159. Li X, Zhang Y, Kang H, Liu W, Liu P, Zhang J, Harris SE, Wu D. Sclerostin binds to LRP5/6 and antagonizes canonical wnt signaling. J Biol Chem. 2005;280:19883–7.
160. Ellies DL, Viviano B, McCarthy J, Rey J-P, Itasaki N, Saunders S, Krumlauf R. Bone density ligand, sclerostin, directly interacts with LRP5 but not LRP5G171V to modulate Wnt activity. J Bone Miner Res. 2006;21:1738–49.
161. Hay E, Bouaziz W, Funck-Brentano T, Cohen-Solal M. Sclerostin and bone aging: a mini-review. Gerontology. 2016;62:618–23.
162. Fang Y, Ginsberg C, Seifert M, Agapova O, Sugatani T, Register TC, Freedman BI, Monier-Faugere M-C, Malluche H, Hruska KA. CKD-induced wingless/integration1 inhibitors and phosphorus cause the CKD-mineral and bone disorder. J Am Soc Nephrol. 2014;25:1760–73.
163. Kanbay M, Siriopol D, Saglam M, et al. Serum sclerostin and adverse outcomes in nondialyzed chronic kidney disease patients. J Clin Endocrinol Metab. 2014;99:E1854–61.
164. García-Martín A, Rozas-Moreno P, Reyes-García R, Morales-Santana S, García-Fontana B, García-Salcedo JA, Muñoz-Torres M. Circulating levels of sclerostin are increased in patients with type 2 diabetes mellitus. J Clin Endocrinol Metab. 2012;97:234–41.
165. Bonani M, Rodriguez D, Fehr T, Mohebbi N, Brockmann J, Blum M, Graf N, Frey D, Wüthrich RP. Sclerostin blood levels before and after kidney transplantation. Kidney Blood Press Res. 2014;39:230–9.
166. Evenepoel P, Claes K, Viaene L, Bammens B, Meijers B, Naesens M, Sprangers B, Kuypers D. Decreased circulating sclerostin levels in renal transplant recipients with persistent hyperparathyroidism. Transplantation. 2016;100:2188–93.
167. Roforth MM, Fujita K, McGregor UI, Kirmani S, McCready LK, Peterson JM, Drake MT, Monroe DG, Khosla S. Effects of age on bone mRNA levels of sclerostin and other genes relevant to bone metabolism in humans. Bone. 2014;59:1–6.
168. Sabbagh Y, Graciolli FG, O'Brien S, et al. Repression of osteocyte Wnt/β-catenin signaling is an early event in the progression of renal osteodystrophy. J Bone Miner Res. 2012;27:1757–72.
169. Cejka D, Herberth J, Branscum AJ, Fardo DW, Monier-Faugere M-C, Diarra D, Haas M, Malluche HH. Sclerostin and Dickkopf-1 in renal osteodystrophy. Clin J Am Soc Nephrol. 2011;6:877–82.
170. Bover J, Ureña P, Brandenburg V, et al. Adynamic bone disease: from bone to vessels in chronic kidney disease. Semin Nephrol. 2014;34:626–40.

171. Moe S, Drüeke T, Cunningham J, Goodman W, Martin K, Olgaard K, Ott S, Sprague S, Lameire N, Eknoyan G. Definition, evaluation, and classification of renal osteodystrophy: a position statement from Kidney Disease: Improving Global Outcomes (KDIGO). Kidney Int. 2006;69:1945–53.

172. Coen G, Mazzaferro S, Ballanti P, Sardella D, Chicca S, Manni M, Bonucci E, Taggi F. Renal bone disease in 76 patients with varying degrees of predialysis chronic renal failure: a cross-sectional study. Nephrol Dial Transpl. 1996;11:813–9.

173. Graciolli FG, Neves KR, Barreto F, et al. The complexity of chronic kidney disease-mineral and bone disorder across stages of chronic kidney disease. Kidney Int. 2017;91:1436–46.

174. Moe SM, Chen NX, Newman CL, Organ JM, Kneissel M, Kramer I, Gattone VH, Allen MR. Anti-sclerostin antibody treatment in a rat model of progressive renal osteodystrophy. J Bone Miner Res. 2015;30:499–509.

175. Gupta A, Kallenbach LR, Zasuwa G, Divine GW. Race is a major determinant of secondary hyperparathyroidism in uremic patients. J Am Soc Nephrol. 2000;11:330–4.

176. Malluche HH, Mawad HW, Monier-Faugere M-C. Renal osteodystrophy in the first decade of the new millennium: analysis of 630 bone biopsies in black and white patients. J Bone Miner Res. 2011;26:1368–76.

177. Cosman F, Morgan DC, Nieves JW, Shen V, Luckey MM, Dempster DW, Lindsay R, Parisien M. Resistance to bone resorbing effects of PTH in black women. J Bone Miner Res. 1997;12:958–66.

178. Fishbane S, Hazzan AD, Jhaveri KD, Ma L, Lacson E. Bone parameters and risk of hip and femur fractures in patients on hemodialysis. Clin J Am Soc Nephrol. 2016;11:1063–72.

179. London GM. Bone-vascular cross-talk. J Nephrol. 2012;25:619–25.

180. London GM, Marty C, Marchais SJ, Guerin AP, Metivier F, de Vernejoul M-C. Arterial calcifications and bone histomorphometry in end-stage renal disease. J Am Soc Nephrol. 2004;15:1943–51.

181. London GM, Marchais SJ, Guerin AP, de Vernejoul MC. Ankle-brachial index and bone turnover in patients on dialysis. J Am Soc Nephrol. 2015;26:476–83.

182. Quarles LD, Lobaugh B, Murphy G. Intact parathyroid hormone overestimates the presence and severity of parathyroid-mediated osseous abnormalities in uremia. J Clin Endocrinol Metab. 1992;75:145–50.

183. Torres A, Lorenzo V, Hernández D, Rodríguez JC, Concepción MT, Rodríguez AP, Hernández A, de Bonis E, Darias E, González-Posada JM. Bone disease in predialysis, hemodialysis, and CAPD patients: evidence of a better bone response to PTH. Kidney Int. 1995;47:1434–42.

184. Hercz G, Pei Y, Greenwood C, Manuel A, Saiphoo C, Goodman WG, Segre GV, Fenton S, Sherrard DJ. Aplastic osteodystrophy without aluminum: the role of suppressed parathyroid function. Kidney Int. 1993;44:860–6.

185. Torregrosa JV, Bover J, Cannata Andia J, et al. Spanish Society of Nephrology recommendations for controlling mineral and bone disorder in chronic kidney disease patients (S.E.N.-M.B.D.). Nefrologia. 2011;31(Suppl 1):3–32.

186. Wein MN. Parathyroid hormone signaling in osteocytes. J Bone Miner Res Plus. 2018;2:22–30.

187. Garrett G, Sardiwal S, Lamb EJ, Goldsmith DJA. PTH—a particularly tricky hormone: why measure it at all in kidney patients? Clin J Am Soc Nephrol. 2013;8:299–312.

188. Yilmaz MI, Siriopol D, Saglam M, et al. Osteoprotegerin in chronic kidney disease: associations with vascular damage and cardiovascular events. Calcif Tissue Int. 2016;99:121–30.

189. DeFronzo RA, Alvestrand A, Smith D, Hendler R, Hendler E, Wahren J. Insulin resistance in uremia. J Clin Invest. 1981;67:563–8.

190. Blum WF, Ranke MB, Kietzmann K, Tönshoff B, Mehls O. Growth hormone resistance and inhibition of somatomedin activity by excess of insulin-like growth factor binding protein in uraemia. Pediatr Nephrol. 1991;5:539–44.

191. Koizumi M, Komaba H, Fukagawa M. Parathyroid function in chronic kidney disease: role of FGF23-Klotho axis. Contrib Nephrol. 2013;180:110–23.
192. Evenepoel P, Rodriguez M, Ketteler M. Laboratory abnormalities in CKD-MBD: markers, predictors, or mediators of disease? Semin Nephrol. 2014;34:151–63.
193. Román-García P, Carrillo-López N, Naves-Díaz M, Rodríguez I, Ortiz A, Cannata-Andía JB. Dual-specificity phosphatases are implicated in severe hyperplasia and lack of response to FGF23 of uremic parathyroid glands from rats. Endocrinology. 2012;153:1627–37.
194. Galitzer H, Ben-Dov IZ, Silver J, Naveh-Many T. Parathyroid cell resistance to fibroblast growth factor 23 in secondary hyperparathyroidism of chronic kidney disease. Kidney Int. 2010;77:211–8.
195. Komaba H, Goto S, Fujii H, et al. Depressed expression of Klotho and FGF receptor 1 in hyperplastic parathyroid glands from uremic patients. Kidney Int. 2010;77:232–8.
196. Brown AJ, Ritter CS, Finch JL, Slatopolsky EA. Decreased calcium-sensing receptor expression in hyperplastic parathyroid glands of uremic rats: role of dietary phosphate. Kidney Int. 1999;55:1284–92.
197. Brown AJ, Dusso A, Lopez-Hilker S, Lewis-Finch J, Grooms P, Slatopolsky E. 1,25-(OH)2D receptors are decreased in parathyroid glands from chronically uremic dogs. Kidney Int. 1989;35:19–23.
198. Mithal A, Kifor O, Kifor I, Vassilev P, Butters R, Krapcho K, Simin R, Fuller F, Hebert SC, Brown EM. The reduced responsiveness of cultured bovine parathyroid cells to extracellular Ca2+ is associated with marked reduction in the expression of extracellular Ca(2+)-sensing receptor messenger ribonucleic acid and protein. Endocrinology. 1995;136:3087–92.
199. Ritter CS, Finch JL, Slatopolsky EA, Brown AJ. Parathyroid hyperplasia in uremic rats precedes down-regulation of the calcium receptor. Kidney Int. 2001;60:1737–44.
200. Fukuda N, Tanaka H, Tominaga Y, Fukagawa M, Kurokawa K, Seino Y. Decreased 1,25-dihydroxyvitamin D3 receptor density is associated with a more severe form of parathyroid hyperplasia in chronic uremic patients. J Clin Invest. 1993;92:1436–43.
201. Silver J, Kilav R, Naveh-Many T. Mechanisms of secondary hyperparathyroidism. Am J Physiol Physiol. 2002;283:F367–76.

PTH Regulation by Phosphate and miRNAs

Antonio Canalejo, Mariano Rodríguez and Yolanda Almadén

Introduction

Beyond the steady rise in the regulating processes being discovered in the last decades for PTH, the far-known canonical function is the minute to minute regulation of extracellular calcium concentrations. Thus, the main natural canonical effector able to regulate parathyroid function, and specifically PTH secretion, is calcium itself. Hypocalcemia sensed trough plasma membrane calcium sensing receptors (CaSR) lead to an increase in PTH release which, in turn, acts on target tissues to restore normal calcium levels. Vitamin D, i.e. calcitriol, the natural active form, by acting through specific intracellular vitamin D receptors (VDR), is also able to regulate PTH synthesis. Hypocalcemia leads to an increase in vitamin D levels to enhance intestinal calcium absorption; then after the calcemia is restored, vitamin D inhibits the PTH synthesis in a safe-guard feedback manner.

This dual calcium-vitamin D model would appear robust enough to cope with the regulation of the parathyroid function. However, compelling clinical and experimental evidences pointed insistently to look at an old well-known key player of the mineral metabolism, phosphate, as a putative new direct effector of the parathyroid glands. But it has resulted highly difficult to state clearly a mechanism of action for the phosphate. In fact, despite the significant efforts made

A. Canalejo
Department of Integrated Sciences/Centro de investigacion RENSMA, University of Huelva, Huelva, Spain

M. Rodríguez (✉)
Instituto Maimónides de Investigación Biomédica de Córdoba (IMIBIC), Reina Sofia University Hospital/University of Córdoba, Córdoba, Spain
e-mail: marianorodriguezportillo@gmail.com

Y. Almadén
Unidad de Gestión Clinica Medicina Interna. Lipid and Atherosclerosis Unit, Department of Internal Medicine/IMIBIC/Reina, Sofia University Hospital/University of Córdoba, CIBER Fisiopatologia Obesidad y Nutricion (CIBEROBN), Instituto de Salud Carlos III, Córdoba, Spain

© Springer Nature Switzerland AG 2020
A. Covic et al. (eds.), *Parathyroid Glands in Chronic Kidney Disease*,
https://doi.org/10.1007/978-3-030-43769-5_5

by researchers to find out a specific phosphate sensor it remained quite elusive. Recent data, however, may be knocking the door to come into the discovery of a receptor able to sense phosphate levels. Furthermore, along the elucidation of the effects of phosphate there was sometimes the perception of being in the foot-steps of a ghost, since the observed alterations in the parathyroid function due to the increase in the phosphate burden was not always associated with an elevation in the serum phosphate levels. And here is where the fibroblast growth factor 23 (FGF23), a phosphatonin that favors renal phosphate excretion, took a preponder-ant role lasting from the last two decades. In part as a surrogate of high phosphate levels with the capacity to be sensed by parathyroid glands through specific recep-tors (a complex of the FGF23 receptor, FGFR1, with the co-receptor α-klotho), but also by targeting other organs involved in the homeostasis of the mineral metabo-lism. This chapter will cover the mechanisms whereby high phosphate modulates the secretion of PTH. And it will also cope with the role of miRNAs, perhaps the last guest star mechanism found to regulate PTH secretion, and which might open new therapeutic prospects.

The Direct Effect of Phosphate on PTH Secretion

From far, clinical and experimental data pointed to phosphate as a modulator of the parathyroid function. Hyperphosphatemia was consistently associated to the production of uremic hyperparathyroidism (secondary hyperparathyroidism, SHPT). Thus, both restriction of dietary phosphorus and chelation of phospho-rus by binders are effective strategies in the prevention and treatment of SHP. However, it was certainly difficult to demonstrate an independent effect of phos-phate on parathyroid cell function, especially in vivo. The beneficial effect of low-ering the phosphate load, e.g. through a low phosphate diet, could be attributed to concomitant changes such as the stimulation of calcitriol production [1–3] and the improvement of hypocalcemia due to an increase in the calcemic response to PTH [3–5]. In an attempt to overcome these physiological constraints, Lopez-Hilker et al. showed that dietary phosphorus restriction improved renal hyperparath-yroidism in dogs independent of changes in calcitriol and serum calcium levels [6]. But, in any case, the undoubted stating of a direct effect of phosphate would require in vitro studies.

Some authors had successfully used rat parathyroid gland in organ culture to test the effect of 1,25-dihydroxyvitamin D, cortisol and calcium on PTH secre-tion [7–9]. However, the first attempts by using parathyroid cell lines or dispersed cells from primary cultures failed to show it. The first study to report a clear direct effect of phosphate on PTH secretion was that of Almaden et al. [10] performed in whole rat parathyroid glands, which was confirmed promptly by other authors in the same model [11]. Then, Nielsen et al. [12] showed this in bovine parathy-roid glands and confirmed that it was only observed in tissue with intact architec-ture. Interestingly, though isolated cells had been shown to be less responsive to changes in extracellular calcium due to a progressive decrease in the expression of the CaSR along the culture time [13–15], both the bovine dispersed cells and tissue preparations responded to changes in the calcium concentration. Furthermore, though an effect of phosphate was observed in dispersed parathyroid cells [16], it was accounted to the presence of cell clusters with close cell-to-cell interaction. To date, however, there is not a clear explanation of why cell-to-cell interaction is important to observe an effect of phosphate on PTH secretion. Sun et al. [17] demonstrated that parathyroid cells in close proximity are stimulated to secrete more PTH and suggest the presence of a paracrine interaction among parathyroid cells. Intercellular communication might be also required to observe an effect of phosphate on PTH secretion. Later studies using a pseudogland model of parathyroid tissue grown in collagen [18] also showed the importance of the 3-D tissue architecture in parathyroid gland function.

The findings by Almaden et al. [10] in normal rat parathyroid glands indicated that a phosphate concentration of 4 or 3 mM increased the basal rate (calcium 1.25 mM) of PTH secretion but it did not increase further the maximal rate of PTH secretion induced by low calcium. Therefore, a high phosphate concentration maintains an abnormally elevated PTH secretion rate despite a normal extracellular calcium level, but it did not further increase PTH secretion when parathyroid glands are maximally stimulated by low extracellular calcium levels. Thus, in vitro, a high phosphate level shifted the PTH-calcium curve to the right, making parathyroid cells less sensitive to inhibition by calcium. This may explain, at least in part, the increase in the set point of the PTH calcium curve observed in hyperphosphatemic patients with uremic hyperparathyroidism.

A later study by Almaden et al. [19] addressed the effect of high phosphate on the secretion of PTH in human hyperplastic parathyroid glands. These parathyroid glands have frequently areas of nodular growth and possess a decreased number of vitamin D and calcium sensor receptors [14, 20]. Thus, they are less responsive to calcium and calcitriol so that the concentration of calcium required to inhibit PTH secretion is greater than normal [21, 22]. Experiments were performed using small pieces of parathyroid glands. In diffuse hyperplastic tissue, a high concentration of phosphate in the incubation media prevented the calcium-induced inhibition of PTH secretion. This effect was more marked with 4 than 3 mM P, suggesting a dose-response effect. In nodular hyperplasia, high phosphate reduced the ability of high calcium to inhibit the PTH secretion; however, the reduction of PTH secretion by calcium was not significantly different between 3 and 1 mM phosphate. Therefore, it was demonstrated in an in vitro setting that high phosphate level stimulates PTH secretion independently of a low calcium concentration and a calcitriol deficiency, which are usually present in uremic patients.

Further demonstration of a direct effect of phosphate on PTH secretion was obtained in in vivo studies in hemodialysis patients [23] and in dogs [24]. Interestingly, these in vivo studies also demonstrated that the effect of phosphate on PTH secretion is dose-dependent; however, the degree of PTH response to phosphate is much lower than to calcium.

The direct stimulatory effect of phosphate on PTH secretion is rapid. In the in vitro setting, it was observed after 2 hours of incubation (unpublished results from our laboratory). In vivo, in uremic rats adapted to a high phosphate diet (HPD), a switch to a meal of low phosphate diet (LPD), caused a decrease in 80% of serum PTH within the 2-hour feeding period with no change in plasma calcium but a 1 mg/dl fall in plasma phosphate [25]. In contrast, HPD gavage increased PTH by 80% within 15 minutes with no change in plasma phosphate or calcium. Furthermore, duodenal and intravenous infusion of sodium phosphate increased PTH within 10 minutes, whereas infusion of sodium chloride had no effect.

Phosphate and PTH Gene Expression

Soon after the demonstration of a direct effect of phosphate on PTH secretion, the search of the underlying molecular mechanisms began. The first issue to be addressed was the possible effect of phosphate on PTH synthesis. In fact, even before the direct effect of phosphate on PTH secretion was uncovered, a number of in vivo studies with different rat models suggested that PTH synthesis was affected by dietary phosphate manipulation in early chronic renal failure [26] and hypophosphatemic rats [27]; a high serum phosphate level was associated with increased PTH mRNA It was also shown that in normal rats a high phosphate diet increased PTH mRNA independent of calcium and CTR levels [28]. Subsequent, in vitro studies with hyperplastic parathyroid tissues from hemodialysis patients showed that the stimulation of PTH secretion by high phosphate levels (4 mM) was accompanied by an increase in PTH mRNA in both diffuse and nodular hyperplasia [19].

In any case, the thorough studies performed by the group of Silver and Naveh-Many along a decade on the regulation of PTH synthesis by calcium and phosphate lead to the conclusion that the effects were post-transcriptional, as shown by nuclear transcript run-on experiments [27, 29, 30]. Thus, calcium and phosphate regulate PTH gene expression by changes in protein-PTH mRNA 3'-untranslated region (UTR) interactions, which determine PTH mRNA stability. By combining in vivo experimental models of hypocalcemic and hypophosphatemic rats with in vitro mRNA degradation assay (IVDA) this group identified both the cis-acting sequences and the trans-acting factors involved in PTH mRNA stabilization and/or decay. There was an approximately 60-fold difference in PTH mRNA levels between hypocalcemic and hypophosphatemic rats.

In a first study, these authors found that a number of parathyroid cytosolic proteins bind to a conserved *cis*-acting element in the parathyroid hormone 3'-UTR [29]; the binding being dependent upon the terminal 60 nucleotides. Parathyroid proteins from hypocalcemic rats showed increased binding and proteins from hypophosphatemic rats showed decreased binding that correlated with PTH mRNA levels. Through IVDA they showed that a PTH mRNA probe maintained intact for 180 minutes after being incubated with cytosolic proteins from hypocalcemic rats but only for 5 minutes in the presence of hypophosphatemic proteins; conversely parathyroid proteins from control rats led the transcript to steady for 40 minutes, while a transcript lacking this region showed no degradation in the presence of hypophosphatemic proteins. Importantly, it was also shown that upon incubation with parathyroid proteins from uremic rats, the PTH mRNA was not degraded at all after 120 min and was moderately decreased at 180 min [30]. Further studies delimited the PTH mRNA-protein binding region to a minimum sequence of 26 nucleotides shown to be necessary and sufficient to confer responsiveness to calcium and phosphate through the regulation of PTH mRNA stability [31].

After the 3′-UTR regulatory region was identified, it was the turn for the specific proteins that bind it. The first was the 50 kDa AU-rich binding (AUF1) protein, which was able to bind to the PTH mRNA 3′-UTR and stabilize the PTH transcript [32]. Interestingly, calcineurin regulates AUF1 post-translationally in vitro and PTH gene expression in vivo but still allows its physiological regulation by calcium and phosphate [33]. The Upstream of N-ras (Unr) protein was shown to be another PTH mRNA 3′-UTR binding protein as part of the parathyroid RNA binding complex [34]. Furthermore, the mRNA decay promoting K-homology splicing regulator protein (KSRP) appeared as a master key in the PTH mRNA post-transcriptional regulatory complex [35]. The binding of KSPR to the 3′-UTR PTH mRNA is decreased in glands from calcium-depleted or experimental chronic kidney failure rats in which PTH mRNA is more stable, compared with parathyroid glands from control and phosphate-depleted rats in which PTH mRNA is less stable. Of note, the activity of KSRP is regulated via its interaction with the peptidyl-prolyl isomerase (PPIase), Pin1, which led to KSRP dephosphorylation and activation [36]. Pin1 activity is decreased in parathyroid protein extracts from both hypocalcemic and CKD rats.

Taken together all these pieces of information, the model whereby phosphate modulates post-transcriptionally the PTH synthesis begins to emerge. Thus, in low serum phosphate conditions active Pin 1 lead to KSRP dephosphorylation and activation, favoring its association with the PTH mRNA 3′-UTR ARE and preventing the binding of the stabilizing complex consisting of AUF1 and Unr. The result is the recruitment of the exosome leading to PTH mRNA decay and then to decreased PTH production [37, 38]. Interestingly, the same mechanism but working in an inverse sense, governs the regulation of PTH gene expression in hypocalcemia and CKD, where Pin 1 activity is reduced favoring the binding of AUF1 and Unr to inhibit PTH mRNA degradation. In any case, this picture still appears incomplete so as it is pending to connect the sensing processes with the regulation of Pin 1 activity and the possible contribution of other new players. Therefore, by contrast to the regulation of PTH synthesis at the transcriptional level defined for the vitamin D, involving the VDR and the VDRE sequences in the *p*th gene, a post-transcriptional mechanism related to cytosolic endonuclease activity, resulting in a more or less stable PTH transcript, appears to account for the effect of calcium and phosphate in the normal and uremic settings. Importantly, this post-transcriptional mechanism appears to be in accordance with the short time taken for the high phosphate levels to increase PTH release.

Searching for a Phosphate Sensor

The way the living organisms cope with phosphate sensing is highly dependent on the compartment in which the phosphate levels must be regulated and thus, two key models are distinguished. The metabolic phosphate sensing functions to maintain levels of phosphate in the intracellular compartment to support cellular metabolism, while the endocrine phosphate sensing drives the homeostatic regulation of phosphate in the extracellular compartment in multicellular organisms [39]. Phosphate sensing mechanism in bacteria and yeast is mainly based on plasma membrane proteins able to modulate phosphate uptake and the activation of signal transduction pathways. Interestingly, metabolic phosphate sensing in multicellular organism as mammals have been also shown to be related to plasma membrane transporters as the type 3 sodium- dependent phosphate transporters PIT1 and/or PIT2, ubiquitous suppliers of phosphate to the cell. However, it has been difficult to identify the endocrine phosphate sensing in mammals [40], which extends to that of parathyroid cell.

Due to the lack of a known specific phosphate sensor in the parathyroid cells that could explain the direct effect of phosphate on the parathyroid function, during the last decades a number of phosphate transporter systems, with a special role for the PIT ones, were proposed to be involved. In fact, a phosphate uptake- independent signaling function of PIT1was reported to be important for VSMC processes mediating vascular calcification [41]. Through this so-called single sensor phosphate hypothesis, the transporter would work together with a co-receptor, as found in the osteocyte to regulate PTH secretion with the participation of FGFR1upon stimulation with phosphate [39]. By the contrary, the so-called multiple sensor hypotheses imply the existence of a second independent sensor, as might be the case for the parathyroids, which has maintained elusive up to now. However, a study by Geng et al. [42] appears to shed new light regarding the phosphate sensing in the parathyroid cells. And, amazingly, it seems to operate at the very core of the regulation of the parathyroid function since it concerns to the CaSR itself. In fact, this outstanding study confirms previous views on this receptor, but also opens new paradigms.

Though extracellular calcium was initially recognized as the specific agonist of the CaSR, it was promptly found out a wide distribution and functional plasticity derived from its ability to bind to other different ligands (including various divalent and trivalent cations, polyamines and cationic polypeptides), and to activate different G proteins-downstream signaling pathways. A main point also came after the demonstration that L-amino acids were allosteric activators able to activate it provided that calcium concentration is above a threshold [43]. Now, as revealed by X-ray crystallography-derived crystal structure of the entire extracellular domain of CaSR in the resting and active conformations, Geng et al. [42] found novel binding sites for calcium, phosphate (PO_4^{3-}) and L-Trp and identified L-Trp as an agonist of the receptor, demonstrating that these ions and amino acids collectively control the function of the CaSR.

The functional CaSR is a disulfide-tethered homodimer composed of three main domains, the Venus Flytrap (VFT) module (that includes two domains, LB1 and LB2), a cysteine-rich domain and the seven-helix transmembrane region. As demonstrated by Geng et al. [42], binding of amino acids, as L-Trp, to specific binding sites facilitates extracellular domain closure of CaSR, a crucial first step during activation, by contacting both LB1 and LB2 domains of the VFT module. Thus, L-Trp directly activates CaSR-mediated intracellular calcium mobilization in the presence of extracellular calcium, which is completely abolishes by the mutation of the L-Trp-binding residues. Therefore, calcium ions are not the main activator of the receptor, since the CaSR maintains an inactive state in the absence or presence of calcium ions, and it is only after the amino acid is bound that the active state forms. Calcium binds to up to four sites with different occupancy and affinity levels resulting in the stabilization of the active conformation of the receptor by facilitating homodimer interactions between the membrane-proximal LB2 and CR domains. Importantly, the effect of amino acids and calcium depends on the each other since a level of calcium is needed for amino acids to activate the CaRS, while this increase its sensitivity toward calcium to gain in stability. Therefore, amino acids appear as orthosteric agonists of CaSR, and they act concertedly with calcium to achieve full receptor activation.

But perhaps the most exciting finding described by Geng et al. [42] concerns to the role of anions on the CaSR function. Contrary to the effect of calcium, phosphate (PO_4^{3-}) reinforce the inactive conformation. They identified a total of four anion-binding sites in the inactive and active structures; sites 1–3 located above the interdomain cleft in the LB1 domain, and site 4 as part of LB2 domain. In the inactive structure, anions bound at sites 1–3 but in the active structure, only sites 2 and 4 are occupied. Binding of phosphate to the active form at site 2 and 4 leads to a negative modulatory effect on the CaSR activity and the concomitant decrease in CaSR-mediated IP accumulation.

All these novel findings depict the functional activity of the CaSR as the result of complex relationships with at least three key ligands to modulate the inactive and active states. In the resting state, L-amino acids induce VFT closure favoring the formation of homodimer interface between subunits, while calcium binding stabilize the active state by enhancing homodimer interactions to fully activate the receptor. By contrast, phosphate binding prevent activation by promoting an inactive configuration. Importantly, these mechanistic findings meet some previous questions as the requirement of a threshold of calcium to observe the effect of phosphate on PTH secretion and previous observations that phosphate makes parathyroid cells less sensitive to inhibition by calcium. And also provide a putative mechanism for the role of polycations as polyamines, which might favor the dissociation of phosphate from the relatively weak anion-binding sites and thus prevent its inhibitory effect. Finally, since the effect of phosphate on the parathyroid cells appears mediated by a cell membrane protein, it may be affected by the tissue digestion required for cell dispersion, which would be the reason of the failure to demonstrate an effect of phosphate on PTH secretion in isolated parathyroid cells.

Regulation of PTH Secretion by miRNAs

MicroRNAs (miRNAs) are small non-coding RNAs involving in post-transcriptional regulation of gene expression. Through interfering RNAs, miRNAs exert a fine-tuning of gene expression and thus contribute as important regulators of numerous physiological and pathological mechanisms. Identification of miRNA functions can indicate novel targets for biological processes and may have significant value as biomarkers of disease etiology and progression [44–46].

The first approximations to study the involvement of miRNAs in the parathyroid cell function were performed in the setting of abnormal parathyroid growth as carcinomas and adenomas. As compared to normal or adenoma tissues, carcinoma tissues showed a specific pattern of *miRNoma* consisting of a set of down-regulated miRNAs as miR-26b, miR-30b, miR-139, miR-126–5p, and miR-296 [47], while others as miR-222, miR-503 and miR-517c appeared up-regulated [48, 49]. As expected, after looking for the putative target genes of these miRNAs, a number of genes related to the regulation of cell growth and malignancy were evidenced. Though undoubtedly this can be related to the regulation of PTH secretion through a role in the development of parathyroid hyperplasia, in the last recent years, two studies by the Naveh-Many's group addressed and uncovered a more direct involvement of miRNAs on PTH secretion [50, 51].

In the first study, Shilo et al. [50] used parathyroid-Dicer$-^{/}-$ mice (unable to produce mature miRNAs in the parathyroid glands) that showed no alterations in the key mineral metabolism parameters since they had normal calcium, phosphate and PTH. When they were subjected to an experimental acute hypocalcemia (by EGTA administration), they failed to show a full increase in PTH as the controls did. Of note, it was also replicated in vitro by incubating the thyroparathyroid glands in a calcium-depleted medium. These authors also demonstrated that a chronic challenge of hypocalcemia, by feeding the parathyroid-Dicer$^{-/-}$ mice with a calcium-depleted diet, resulted in a much-reduced increase in PTH, one third of the response observed in the control mice; and, importantly, there was no increase in PTH mRNA. Also, of special interest is that, by contrast to what it happened in the controls, there was no stimulation of parathyroid proliferation in the defective animals. Finally, Shilo et al. [50] evaluated these events in the setting of a rat model of uremia and SHP induced by an adenine high phosphate diet. In spite of having similar levels of uremia, again the uremic counterparts failed to increase PTH to the same extent as in the control mice (in a two to four-fold relationship), as well as the parathyroid proliferation. However, it was extremely interesting that when they assessed the response of the parathyroid-Dicer$-^{/}-$ mice to a hypercalcemic challenge (by an i.v. injection of calcium gluconate), they found a normal inhibition of PTH secretion, similar to that of controls. And it was correspondingly replicated after treatment with calcimimetic. These comprehensive results showed that the normal response of parathyroid glands to both hypocalcemia (acute and chronic) and uremia (involving induction of PTH secretion and proliferation) is dependent on the dicer activity and, then of specific miRNAs. The conserved

CaSR sensitivity to hypercalcemia of PT-Dicer1$^{-/-}$ cells indicates that the parathyroid functions related to the gene expression/activation of the CaSR appears not to be under the regulation by miRNAs.

In a second significant study, Shilo et al. [51] first profiled miRNAs in normal mouse, rat and human parathyroid glands by small-RNA sequencing. They found conservation of expression of miRNAs among species; among the 50 most abundant sequence families in human parathyroid, 37 were also top 50 in mouse and 39 in rat. let-7 members were the most highly expressed ranging 23–32% and then the miR-30 (8.9–14%) and miR-141/200 members (4.5–8.5%). These similar profiles of abundant miRNAs, suggest an evolutionarily conserved regulation of functions in parathyroid physiology. Then, these authors studied the function of some of these specific miRNAs in parathyroid glands from patients receiving dialysis and from experimental uremic models of SHP as a short-term uremia (induced by 1-week adenine diet with high-phosphate content), an intermediate/long-term uremia (6–8 weeks of the diet), and a hypocalcemia (induced by a 3-week feeding with a low-calcium content diet). As compared to the normal glands, mayor *miRNome* alterations were found. Of the six most abundant miRNAs families in rat parathyroid, four families (miR-30, miR-148, miR-141, and miR-21) were significantly up-regulated in SHP, whereas two (let-7 and miR-375) were no significantly down-regulated. Interestingly, while some miRNAs alterations were shared by all SPH models, other specific patterns were dependent on the cause of SHP. And, of note, in a dose-response manner, the more severe the experimental SHP was, the more outlying the miRNAs profiles were. Thus, miRNAs families were gradually up-regulated or down-regulated following a progressive trend from the early CKD to the hypocalcemia (as an intermediate CKD) and then to the late CKD.

Then, Shilo et al. [51] studied the effect of inhibiting specific miRNAs, as the abundant let-7 family, by injecting antagonizing oligonucleotides twice weekly for 4 weeks. Treatment with anti–let-7 oligonucleotides increased serum PTH in both normal and CKD rats. In accordance, let-7 anti-miRNAs added to the growth medium of mouse thyro-parathyroid organ cultures increased PTH secretion. Thus, the let-7 family members were suggested to regulate PTH by restraining PTH production or secretion. By contrast, administration of anti–miR-148 led to significant decrease in serum PTH in the CKD rats, which also was corroborated in vitro in parathyroids from CKD mice; thus, indicating that the miR-148 members promote PTH secretion.

Undoubtedly, these pioneer studies ascertaining the contribution of specific miRNAs in PTH secretion throughout the SHP pathogenesis are just opening a hopeful future in that they can be manipulated to potentially manage the disease. In fact, it is already being extending to other related branches of the disease. Thus, as compared to healthy controls, in patients with CKD stage 4 and 5 there was a downregulation of miR-223-3p and miR-93-5p, which were associated with CKD stages, parameters of vascular calcification, inflammation and kidney function [52]. Interestingly, a trend towards an association with PTH was also seen. Furthermore, this down-regulation disappeared after kidney transplantation even when lower glomerular filtration rates persisted. In another study, vascular smooth muscle-specific miR-143 and miR-145 expressions were decreased while that of miR-126 was markedly increased, all of them regulating the expression of protein targets involved in vascular alteration associated with CKD [44]. Therefore, miR-NAs appear as new players in the CKD-MBD field [45] that might be of help to assess changes and to prevent or treat complications of CKD as the vascular risk in these patients.

References

1. Portale AA, Halloran BP, Murphy MM, Morris RC Jr. Oral intake of phosphorus can determine the serum concentration of 1,25-dihydroxyvitamin D by determining its production rate in humans. J Clin Invest. 1986;77:7–12.
2. Portale AA, Halloran B. Morris Jr RC Physiologic regulation of serum concentration of 1,25-dihydroxyvitamin D by phosphorus in normal men. J Clin Invest. 1989;83:1494–9.
3. Llach F, Massry SG. On the mechanism of secondary hyperparathyroidism in moderate renal failure. J Clin Endocrinol Metab. 1985;61:601–6.
4. Somerville PJ. Kayc M Evidence that resistance to the calcemic action of parathyroid hormone in rats with acute uremia is caused by phosphate retention. Kidney Int. 1979;16:552–60.
5. Rodriguez M, Martin-Malo A, Martinez ME, Torres A, Felscnfeld AJ, Llach F. Calcemic response to parathyroid hormone in renal failure: Role of phosphorus and its effect on calcitriol. Kidney Int. 1991;40:1055–62.
6. Lopez-Hilker S, Dusso AS, Rapp NS, Martin KJ, Slatopolsky E. Phosphorus restriction reverses hyperparathyroidism in uremia independent of changes in calcium and CTR. Am J Physiol. 1990;259:F432–7.
7. Au WYW, Poland AP, Stern PH. Raisz LG Hormone synthesis and secretion by parathyroid glands in tissue culture. J Clin Invest. 1970;49:1639–46.
8. Au WYW. Cortisol stimulation of parathyroid hormone secretion by rat parathyroid glands in organ culture. Science. 1976;193:1015–7.
9. Au WYW. Inhibition of 1,25 Dihydroxicholecalciferol of hormonal secretion of rat parathyroid gland in organ culture. Calcif Tissue Int. 1984;36:384–91.
10. Almaden Y, Canalejo A, Hernandez A, Ballesteros E, Garcia-Navarro S, Torres A, Rodriguez M. Direct effect of phosphorus on PTH secretion from whole rat parathyroid gland in vitro. J Bone Min Res. 1996;11:970–6.
11. Slatopolsky E, Finch J, Denda M, Ritter C, Zhong M, Dusso A, MacDonald P, Brown A. Phosphorus restriction prevents parathyroid gland growth. High phosphate directly stimulates PTH secretion in vitro. J Clin Invest. 1996;97:2534–40.
12. Nielsen PK, Feldt-Rasmussen U, Olgaard K. A direct effect in vitro of phosphate on PTH release from bovine parathyroid tissue slices but not from dispersed parathyroid cells. Nephrol Dial Transplant. 1996;11:1762–8.
13. Brown AJ, Ritter CS, Finch JL, Slatopolsky EA. Decreased calcium-sensing receptor expression in hyperplastic parathyroid glands of uremic rats: role of dietary phosphate. Kidney Int. 1999;55:1284–92.
14. Kifor O, Moore FD Jr, Wang P, Goldstein M, Vassilev P, Kifor I, Hebert SC, Brown EM. Reduced immunostaining for the extracellular Ca+− sensing receptor in primary and uremic secondary hyperparathyroidism. J Clin Endocrinol Metab. 1996;8:1598–606.
15. Gogusev J, Duchambon P, Hory B, Giovannini M, Goureau Y, Sarfati E, Drüeke TB. Depressed expression of calcium receptor in parathyroid gland tissue of patients with hyperparathyroidism. Kidney Int. 1997;51:328–36.

16. Roussanne MC, Gogusev J, Hory B, Duchambon P, Souberbielle JC, Nabarra B, Pierrat D, Sarfati E, Drueke T, Bourdeau A. Persistence of Ca2+− sensing receptor expression in functionally active, long-term human parathyroid cell cultures. J Bone Miner Res. 1998;13:354–62.

17. Sun F, Maercklein P and Fitzpatrick LA: Paracrine interactions among parathyroid cells. Effect of cell density on cell secretion. J Bone Miner Res. 1994;9: 971–6.

18. Ritter CS, Slatopolsky E, Santoro S, Brown AJ. Parathyroid cells cultured in collagen matrix retain calcium responsiveness: importance of three-dimensional tissue architecture. J Bone Miner Res. 2004;19:491–8.

19. Almaden Y, Hernandez A, Torregrosa V, Canalejo A, Sabate L, Fernandez Cruz L, Campistol JM, Torres A, Rodriguez M. High phosphate level directly stimulates parathyroid hormone secretion and synthesis by human parathyroid tissue in vitro. J Am Soc Nephrol. 1998;9:1845–52.

20. Fukuda N, Tanaka H, Tominaga Y, Fukagawa M, Kurokawa K, Seino Y. Decreased 1,25-dihydroxyvitamin D3 receptor density is associated with a more severe form of parathyroid hyperplasia in chronic uremic patients. J Clin Invest. 1993;92:1436–43.

21. Brown EM. Four-parameter model of the sigmoidal relationship between parathyroid hormone release and extracellular calcium concentration in normal and abnormal parathyroid tissue. J Clin Endocrinol Metab. 1983;56:572–81.

22. Wallfelt C, Gylfe E, Larsson R, Ljunghall S, Rastad J, Akerström G. Relationship between external and cytoplasmic calcium concentrations, parathyroid hormone release and weight of parathyroid glands in human hyperparathyroidism. J Endocrinol. 1988;116:457–64.

23. de Francisco ALM, Cobo MA, Setien MA, Rodrigo E, Frsenedo GF, Unzueta MT, Amado JA, Ruiz JC, Arias M, Rodriguez M. Effect of serum phosphate on parathyroid hormone secretion during hemodialysis. Kidney Int. 1995;54:2140–5.

24. Estepa JC, Aguilera-Tejero E, Lopez I, Almaden Y, Rodriguez M, Felsenfeld AJ. Effect of phosphate on PTH secretion in vivo. J Bone Min Res. 1999;14:1848–54.

25. Martin DR, Ritter CS, Slatopolsky E, Brown AJ. Acute regulation of parathyroid hormone by dietary phosphate. Am J Physiol Endocrinol Metab. 2005;289:E729–34.

26. Yi H, Fukagawa M, Yamato H, Kumagai M, Watanabe T, Kurokawa K. Prevention of enhanced parathyroid hormone secretion, synthesis and hyperplasia by mild dietary phosphorus restriction in early chronic renal failure in rats: possible direct role of phosphorus. Nephron. 1995;70:242–8.

27. Kilav R, Silver J, Naveh-Many T. Parathyroid hormone gene expression in hypophosphatemic rats. J Clin Invest. 1995;96:327–33.

28. Hernández A, Concepción MT, Rodríguez M, Salido E, Torres A. High phosphorus diet increases preproPTH mRNA independent of calcium and calcitriol in normal rats. Kidney Int. 1996;50:1872–8.

29. Moallem E, Kilav R, Silver J, Naveh-Many T. RNA-Protein binding and post-transcriptional regulation of parathyroid hormone gene expression by calcium and phosphate. J Biol Chem. 1998;273:5253–9.

30. Yalcindag C, Silver J, Naveh-Many T. Mechanism of increased parathyroid hormone mRNA in experimental uremia: roles of protein RNA binding and RNA degradation. J Am Soc Nephrol. 1999;10:2562–8.

31. Kilav R, Bell O, Le SY, Silver J, Naveh-Many T. The parathyroid hormone mRNA 3′-untranslated region AU-rich element is an unstructured functional element. J Biol Chem. 2004;279:2109–16.

32. Sela-Brown A, Silver J, Brewer G, Naveh-Many T. Identification of AUF1 as a parathyroid hormone mRNA 3′-untranslated region-binding protein that determines parathyroid hormone mRNA stability. J Biol Chem. 2000;275:7424–9.

33. Bell O, Gaberman E, Kilav R, Levi R, Cox KB, Molkentin JD, Silver J, Naveh-Many T. The protein phosphatase calcineurin determines basal parathyroid hormone gene expression. Mol Endocrinol. 2005;19:516–26.

34. Dinur M, Kilav R, Sela-Brown A, Jacquemin-Sablon H, Naveh-Many T. In vitro evidence that upstream of N-ras participates in the regulation of parathyroid hormone messenger ribonucleic acid stability. Mol Endocrinol. 2006;20:1652–60.

35. Nechama M, Ben-Dov IZ, Briata P, Gherzi R, Naveh-Many T. The mRNA decay promoting factor K-homology splicing regulator protein post-transcriptionally determines parathyroid hormone mRNA levels. FASEB J. 2008;22:3458–68. https://doi.org/10.1096/fj.08-107250.

36. Nechama M, Uchida T, Mor Yosef-Levi I, Silver J, Naveh-Many T. The peptidyl-prolyl isomerase Pin1 determines parathyroid hormone mRNA levels and stability in rat models of secondary hyperparathyroidism. J Clin Invest. 2009;119:3102–14. https://doi.org/10.1172/JCI39522.

37. Silver J, Naveh-Many T. Phosphate and the parathyroid. Kidney Int. 2009;75:898–905. https://doi.org/10.1038/ki.2008.642.

38. Naveh-Many T. Minireview: The play of proteins on the parathyroid hormone messenger ribonucleic Acid regulates its expression. Endocrinology. 2010;151:1398–402. https://doi.org/10.1210/en.2009-1160.

39. Chande S, Bergwitz C. Role of phosphate sensing in bone and mineral metabolism. Nat Rev Endocrinol. 2018;14:637–55. https://doi.org/10.1038/s41574-018-0076-3.

40. Sabbagh, Y. Phosphate as a sensor and signaling molecule. Clin Nephrol. 2013;79:57–65. https://doi.org/10.5414/CN107322.

41. Chavkin NW, Chia JJ, Crouthamel MH, Giachelli CM. Phosphate uptake- independent signaling functions of the type III sodium-dependent phosphate transporter, PiT-1, in vascular smooth muscle cells. Exp Cell Res. 2015;333:39–48. https://doi.org/10.1016/j.yexcr.2015.02.002.

42. Geng Y, Mosyak L, Kurinov I, Zuo H, Sturchler E, Cheng TC, Subramanyam P, Brown AP, Brennan SC, Mun HC, Bush M, Chen Y, Nguyen TX, Cao B, Chang DD, Quick M, Conigrave AD, Colecraft HM, McDonald P, Fan QR. Structural mechanism of ligand activation in human calcium-sensing receptor. eLife. 2016;5:e13662. https://doi.org/10.7554/eLife.13662.

43. Conigrave AD, Mun HC, Delbridge L, Quinn SJ, Wilkinson M, Brown EM. L-amino acids regulate parathyroid hormone secretion. J Biol Chem. 2004;279:38151–9. https://doi.org/10.1074/jbc.M406373200.

44. Taïbi F, Metzinger-Le Meuth V, M'Baya-Moutoula E, Djelouat MS, Louvet L, Bugnicourt JM, Poirot S, Bengrine A, Chillon JM, Massy ZA, Metzinger L. Possible involvement of microRNAs in vascular damage in experimental chronic kidney disease. Biochim Biophys Acta. 2014;1842:88–98. https://doi.org/10.1016/j.bbadis.2013.10.005.

45. Metzinger-Le Meuth V, Burtey S, Maitrias P, Massy ZA, Metzinger L. microRNAs in the pathophysiology of CKD-MBD: Biomarkers and innovative drugs. Biochim Biophys Acta Mol Basis Dis. 2017;1863:337–45. https://doi.org/10.1016/j.bbadis.2016.10.027.

46. Jeong S, Oh JM, Oh KH, Kim IW. Differentially expressed miR-3680-5p is associated with parathyroid hormone regulation in peritoneal dialysis patients. PLoS One. 2017;12:e0170535. https://doi.org/10.1371/journal.pone.0170535.

47. Rahbari R, Holloway AK, He M, Khanafshar E, Clark OH, Kebebew E. Identification of differentially expressed MicroRNA in parathyroid tumors. Ann Surg Oncol. 2011;18:1158–65. https://doi.org/10.1245/s10434-010-1359-7.

48. Corbetta S, Vaira V, Guarnieri V, Scillitani A, Eller-Vainicher C, Ferrero S, Vicentini L, Chiodini I, Bisceglia M, Beck-Peccoz P, Bosari S, Spada A. Differential expression of microRNAs in human parathyroid carcinomas compared with normal parathyroid tissue. Endocr Relat Cancer. 2010;17:135–46. https://doi.org/10.1677/ERC-09-0134.

49. Vaira V, Verdelli C, Forno I, Corbetta S. MicroRNAs in parathyroid physiopathology. Mol Cell Endocrinol. 2017;456:9–15. https://doi.org/10.1016/j.mce.2016.10.035.

50. Shilo V, Ben-Dov IZ, Nechama M, Silver J, Naveh-Many T. Parathyroid-specific deletion of dicer-dependent microRNAs abrogates the response of the parathyroid to acute and

chronic hypocalcemia and uremia. FASEB J. 2015;29:3964–76. https://doi.org/10.1096/fj.15-274191.

51. Shilo V, Mor-Yosef Levi I, Abel R, Mihailović A, Wasserman G, Naveh-Many T, Ben-Dov IZ. *Let-7* and *MicroRNA-148* regulate parathyroid hormone levels in secondary hyperparathyroidism. J Am Soc Nephrol. 2017;28:2353–63. https://doi.org/10.1681/ASN.2016050585.

52. Ulbing M, Kirsch AH, Leber B, Lemesch S, Münzker J, Schweighofer N, Hofer D, Trummer O, Rosenkranz AR, Müller H, Eller K, Stadlbauer V, Obermayer-Pietsch B. MicroRNAs 223-3p and 93-5p in patients with chronic kidney disease before and after renal transplantation. Bone. 2017;95:115–23. https://doi.org/10.1016/j.bone.2016.11.016.

PTH Measurement in CKD

Etienne Cavalier

Introduction

Parathormone (PTH), together with 1,25(OH)2 vitamin D, plays a key role in the phosphocalcic regulation. PTH acts primarily on kidney and bone where it binds to cells expressing the type 1 PTH/PTHrP receptor (PTH1R), a G-protein coupled receptor of 1078 amino acids which consists of a large amino-terminal extracellular domain, seven transmembrane helical domains and an intracellular C-tail segment [1]. The very first N-terminal amino-acids of the PTH molecule are indispensable for this interaction [2]. In the kidney, PTH stimulates the reabsorption of calcium in the distal tubule and the activity of the 1-alpha hydroxylase in the renal proximal tubule, thus enhancing the synthesis of 1,25(OH)2 vitamin D. This active metabolite of vitamin D increases the intestinal absorption of calcium and exerts an endocrine feed-back on the secretion of the peptide. PTH also decreases the renal reabsorption of phosphate in the proximal tubule through the endocytosis of the apical sodium dependent cotransporter Npt2a [3]. At longer term, PTH induces changes in Ca metabolism by its action on osteoblasts and indirectly on osteoclasts.

Besides bone, PTH also acts on other different tissues including brain, heart, smooth muscles, lungs, erythrocytes, lymphocytes, pancreas, adrenal glands, testes and motoneural conduction. Since increasing levels of PTH in CKD can have a negative impact on these cells, PTH is thus considered as a uremic toxin [4, 5]. These actions can classically occur through the PTH1R, but a second PTH receptor, called PTH2R, is also expressed in the central nervous system, thyroid, gastrointestinal tract, pancreatic islet cells, and the cardiovascular system, but not in renal tubules.

E. Cavalier (✉)
Department of Clinical Chemistry, University of Liege, CHU de Liege,
Domaine du Sart-Tilman, 4000 Liège, Belgium
e-mail: Etienne.cavalier@chuliege.be

© Springer Nature Switzerland AG 2020
A. Covic et al. (eds.), *Parathyroid Glands in Chronic Kidney Disease*,
https://doi.org/10.1007/978-3-030-43769-5_6

Synthesis, Metabolization of PTH and PTH Fragments

The human PTH gene is located on the short arm of chromosome 11 [6]. The peptide is formed in the chief cells of the parathyroid glands as a large polypeptide that then undergoes two successive proteolytic cleavages to yield PTH, the principal form of the hormone stored in and secreted from the glands. Once secreted, half-life of PTH is of 2–4 minutes. Its metabolization is performed through uptake by the liver and kidneys, which release amino- and carboxy-terminal fragments [7]. PTH degradation also occurs in the parathyroid glands itself, when the calcium-sensing receptor (CaSR) becomes saturated, in cases of high calcium concentration. Low extracellular calcium promotes the release of (1–84) PTH in the circulation. However, when the CaSR is activated by circulating elevated Ca^{++} levels, it causes the release of intracellular Ca in the parathyroid cells, which in turn inhibits the secretion of PTH (1–84) in the circulation. This inhibition is accompanied by an enhanced proteolysis of the NH2-terminal part of the PTH peptide. This degradation process leads to the production of large C-terminal fragments (generally called "non-(1–84) PTH" or "(7–84) PTH"), which have a higher half-live than (1–84) PTH [8]. They also accumulate in the blood of patients suffering from CKD [9]. These fragments are not only a degradation product of PTH and are also secreted by the parathyroid glands [8]. In normal individuals, they account for 15–30% of the total PTH, but in CKD patients, this percentage can be as high as 70–80%.

Preanalytical Considerations in PTH Testing

PTH Stability

The best sample to use for PTH determination, EDTA or plain tubes, as well as sample handling and storage conditions is an important matter of controversy. The advantages of using EDTA over plain tubes (or the opposite) have been described in [10]. Briefly, EDTA tubes allow some time saving in the pre-treatment of samples since it is not necessary to wait a complete coagulation of the samples before centrifugation. Also, EDTA prevents from coagulation-induced interferences and allows a higher yield of sample volume compared to serum. On the other hand, addition of anticoagulants or the presence of fibrinogen may interfere with some analytical methods and concomitant measurement of calcium (which is mandatory for a correct interpretation of PTH levels) or (bone) alkaline phosphatase will need a second tube if EDTA is used. Hence, stability of PTH in EDTA or plain tubes could be a major driver to decipher which tube should be used. Many different publications and a systematic review [11] have been published about PTH stability in EDTA and gel serum tubes. However, the results of these studies are discrepant, mainly due to the variability of their design or on the definition of stability. What can be summarized form these studies is that PTH is more stable in EDTA than in serum gel tubes, especially if samples have to remain unprocessed at room temperature. If the samples can be processed rapidly, serum gel tubes can be recommended, since they offer the advantage of the concomitant determination of calcium and (bone) alkaline phosphatase [12]. Very few studies have correctly evaluated long-term PTH stability at $-20\,°C$ or $-80\,°C$ and, again, these studies used different protocols, complicating the interpretation of the results obtained. Basically, we can summarize that PTH seems stable for 1 year in serum and plasma, at $-20\,°C$ or $-80\,°C$.

Other Preanalytical Variables

Sampling Site

In clinical practice, samples for PTH determination are generally obtained from the antecubital vein, but in hemodialysis patients, samples are frequently taken through the central venous catheter line or the arteriovenous fistula. Since results may significantly differ between peripheral and central sites of sampling [13], the IFCC Working Group on PTH strongly recommends that blood samples for PTH measurement should always be collected from the same sample site for comparison both within and between individuals [11].

Sampling Time

About 20 studies (reviewed in [11]) have evaluated the circadian rhythm of PTH and most of them show a bimodal rhythm, with a nocturnal acrophase, a morning nadir and an afternoon peak. These studies also show considerable intra-individual variability in the circadian fashion. Since the PTH nadir of all these studies is approximately at the same period of time—grossly between 08:00 and 10:00 AM for most of them—and because calcium contained in the diet can influence the PTH concentration, we recommend that PTH is measured in a fasting status in the morning, even if the literature reports conflicting results on the impact of food intake on PTH concentrations. This is in contradiction with the IFCC working group that (weakly) recommends that samples should be collected between 10:00 and 16:00. In hemodialyzed patients, samples should be always taken at the same time, and the fasting status is not mandatory. Finally, PTH is secreted in a tonic fashion, with about 25% of the peptide secreted as small amplitude pulses, around three times an hour [14]. This can contribute to the relatively important intra-individual variation of PTH and should be taken into consideration when interpreting PTH results.

Seasonal Variation

PTH concentrations follow a seasonal variation (lower in summer, higher in winter), probably mirroring the fluctuations of 25(OH)-vitamin D levels. In growing male adolescents, PTH values were 25% lower in summer [15] whereas in patients suffering from primary hyperparathyroidism, this decrease was of 11% [16] (both p<0.0001). Of note, patients taking vitamin D supplements do not present this variation anymore [17]. This finding is important when establishing reference ranges for PTH. Indeed, as recommended in the Guidelines for the management of asymptomatic primary hyperparathyroidism, PTH reference ranges should be established in vitamin D replete patients, with serum concentration of 25(OH)-vitamin D >30 ng/ml [18].

Analytical Considerations

PTH Generation Assays

The description of the first immunoassay for parathyroid hormone was published by Berson and Yalow in 1963 [19]. In the early seventies, many laboratories used to perform PTH determination with what we call now the "first generation" assays. These radio-immunoassays (RIA assays) used a single anti-PTH antibody targeted against the C-terminal part of the peptide and a ^{125}I labelled peptide (generally from bovine origin). Seven days were generally needed to obtain a result.

These assays suffered from important interferences due to the C-terminal fragments, which was especially important in hemodialyzed patients. In 1987, Nichols launched an Immunoradiometric (IRMA) kit called "Allegro" [20]. This immunoradiometric assay used a pair of different antibodies: a capture antibody coated to a plastic bead was directed against the (39–84) portion of the PTH molecule, and a ^{125}I labelled antibody recognized the (13–24) portion of the peptide. This "sandwich" assay was thus not influenced any more by the C-terminal or mid-fragments which were measured with the first-generation assays. This "second-generation" assay kit and the ones that followed were globally called "intact" PTH assays as they were thought to measure only the full-length (1–84) PTH. During the following years, several similar assays, either IRMA or fully automated chemiluminescent assays have become available on the market. Some of them use an anti-N-terminal antibody directed, like the Allegro assay, towards the proximal (13–24) portion of the hormone, whereas others, like Roche Elecsys intact PTH assay, recognize a more distal epitope, in the (26–32) portion.

Even if these second generation kits gave results much more consistent with the clinic, they were rapidly shown to present some limitations. Indeed, several reports suggested that they overestimated the degree of secondary hyperparathyroidism in CRF patients, with some patients presenting elevated "intact" PTH concentrations whereas they presented histological features of low turnover bone disease [21, 22]. These apparent discrepancies were explained in 1998, after the demonstration that several "intact" PTH assays recognized, with various cross-reactivities (from approximately 50% to 100%), a PTH molecule different from the (1–84) PTH, which co-eluted in HPLC with a synthetic (7–84) PTH fragment [23]. This fraction was then called the "non-(1–84) PTH" or, by extension, "(7–84) PTH".

In 1999, the first "third-generation" PTH assay was developed by Scantibodies Laboratories [24]. This IRMA, called "Whole PTH assay" or "Bio-intact PTH", uses an anti-C-terminal antibody similar to those of the "intact" PTH assays, but an anti-N-terminal antibody directed against the very first amino-acids of the peptide (1–4). Thus, this IRMA does not measure the "non-1–84" PTH fragments anymore. Automated methods are now also available for the measurement of 3rd generation PTH on different platforms.

PTH Standardization

PTH assays are not yet standardized and this has an important impact on the inter-analytical methods variability since different assays will produce different results. For this purpose, an IFCC working group on PTH standardization has been created in 2010. The WG has published in 2017 the perspectives and priorities for improvement of PTH measurement [25]. According to the results of PTH (1–84) recovery, it is clear that if all PTH methods were calibrated against the same material, between-method agreement would improve. Hence, the WG has proposed the use of a single international recognized standard "such as" WHO PTH IS 95/646. This standard is composed of recombinant human Parathyroid hormone 1–84 and comes in ampoules that contain 100 µg of PTH 1–84. However, this standard cannot be imposed yet because its commutability must be formally assessed beforehand. Also, a candidate reference measurement procedure for PTH determination does not exist yet. To date, two LCMS/MS have been published so far [26, 27], but they lack sensitivity and reproducibility still need to be demonstrated. PTH standardization will be one of the most important challenges of the newly formed IFCC Committee Bone metabolism. If standardization of all PTH assays can theoretically be achieved in non-CKD patients, this will be impossible for CKD ones. Indeed, as long as GFR decreases, PTH fragments start to accumulate. These fragments are recognized, at different extents, with the antibodies used in the 2nd generation ("intact") PTH assays present on the market. Hence, the standardization will be lost with these methods and only 3rd generation PTH assays can thus be completely standardized in all the populations.

Oxydized PTH

PTH peptide possesses two methionines, one on position 8 and the other on position 18. These methionines are prone to be oxidized, especially in HD patients who suffer from a very intense oxidative stress [28]. Many studies, mainly from the eighties, have shown that oxidized PTH was inactive: it has a lower binding affinity to the PTH receptor and, when bound to the receptor, is unable to generate cAMP; it loses its biological action on smooth muscle cells, cannot stimulate alkaline phosphatase activity in neonatal bone cells and, finally, cannot regulate calcium and phosphate metabolisms in different animal models [29]. Immunoassays for PTH recognize both the oxidized and non-oxidized forms, and the only way to measure to non-oxidized form is to perform a chromatography on an affinity column with fixed antibodies that selectively capture oxidized PTH, allowing then to measure the non-oxidized PTH with any PTH assay. It seems however that the antibodies used in the different PTH assays present different recognize at different extents the oxidized PTH due to difference in cross-reactivities (or matrix effect) [30]. Also, an important question to solve is to know whether or not PTH oxidation occurs in vivo or in vitro. A recent study has indirectly answer the question by proving that non-oxidized PTH was stable in EDTA plasma and that oxidation did not occur after 180 minutes until centrifugation [30]. A fourth generation PTH assay, fully standardized, that would easily measure the non-oxidized (1–84) PTH might thus be of interest. Indeed, a study has demonstrated that patients in the highest versus the lowest non-oxidized PTH tertile presented increased survival and that higher non-oxidized PTH reduced the odds for death [31]. These data were confirmed in patients from the EVOLVE trial: non-oxidized PTH, but not oxidized or intact PTH, had a predictive value for cardiovascular events and all-cause mortality (data not yet published, but presented as a poster at the 2014 ASN by Hocher et al.). These results were infirmed in a cohort of patients with CKD presenting a e-GFR range between 89 and 15 ml/min/1.73 m^2 [32], but this negative finding might be attributable to the fact that these patients were non hemodialyzed. Indeed, HD patients present a much more intensive oxidative stress compared to non-HD CKD patients.

Post-analytical Considerations

Biological Variability and Least Significant Change

Biological variability is of paramount importance to define optimal, desirable and minimal bias and coefficient of variation of analytical methods, which allows calculating allowable total error. It is also largely used to calculate the least significant change, namely the minimal percentage of variation between two successive results that is considered as biologically significant. Establishment of intra- and inter-individual variability (CVw and CVg) is very complicated and most of laboratorians refer to the Westgard website that presents a desirable biological variation database (https://www.westgard.com/biodatabase1.htm). From this website, one can see that CVw and CVg for PTH in plasma is 25.3 and 43.4%, respectively, whereas it is of 25.9 and 23.8% in serum, respectively. These data are based on two papers published in 2008, one from Viljoen et al. [33] and the second by Ankrah-Tetteh et al. [34]. Since 2008, other papers have evaluated the biological variation of PTH, in healthy subjects and hemodialyzed patients and the results show that CVw are very similar between healthy subjects and hemodialyzed patients whereas CVg is much higher in patients, which is logical. From these data, we can calculate that the LSC is around 60% for both patients and subjects. These results have important clinical and analytical implications. From a clinical perspective, a LSC at 60% means that there is no significant biological change in a patient or a subject's PTH result if the increase (or decrease) is not higher than 60%. If we consider a subject with a previous PTH value at 50 ng/L (the upper reference range of the 2nd generation Roche PTH assay), a significant change in his PTH concentration will be considered as biologically significant if is higher than 30 ng/L i.e. if the subject presents a PTH higher than 80 ng/L or lower than 20 ng/L. In the same vein, a PTH change in a hemodialyzed patient that presented a PTH at 300 ng/L will be considered as significant if it is higher or lower than 180 ng/L (>480 or <120 ng/L). This is one of the reasons why the KDIGO guidelines insist on the trend of PTH variation instead of taking a single value into consideration.

Reference Range

In hemodialyzed patients, KDIGO guidelines recommend to maintain the serum PTH levels within twice to 9 times the upper normal limit of the reference range [35]. Accordingly, the definition of the upper limit of the PTH normal range is of prime importance. This raises the question of the inclusion/exclusion criteria which should be applied when recruiting a reference population to establish PTH normal values. Exclusion criteria for this population can be defined as any situation possibly inducing an increase or a decrease in PTH concentration. Among these conditions, low serum 25-hydroxyvitamin D (25OHD) concentration is highly frequent in the general population [36] and should thus be prevalent in an apparently healthy group recruited to establish normal PTH values. Excluding subjects with vitamin D insufficiency from a reference population for serum PTH reference values seems thus logical and has been strongly recommended in the two most recent guidelines on the diagnosis and management of asymptomatic PHPT [18]. We have also demonstrated in several studies that excluding subjects with a low serum 25OHD concentration from a reference population decreased the upper normal limit for serum PTH by 20–35%, depending on the assay considered [37, 38]. Besides 25(OH)D levels, renal function should also be taken into consideration when establishing PTH reference values. Indeed, PTH generally rises when estimated glomerular filtration rate (eGFR) is below 60 mL/min/1.73 m^2. As a decreased renal function may be present, but ignored, in some apparently healthy subjects (especially in those aged more than 60 years) a creatinine measurement to determine the eGFR is mandatory when establishing reference ranges. Other parameters like age, BMI, dietary calcium intakes and ethnicity may also influence PTH reference ranges and further studies are need to determine whether reference PTH values should be stratified according to some of these parameters. We have shown that using PTH reference ranges established according to these criteria clearly improved the KDGO classification of the patients [38].

References

1. Ramasamy I. Inherited disorders of calcium homeostasis. Clin Chim Acta [Internet]. 2008 Aug 1 [cited 2018 Jul 9];394(1–2):22–41. Retrieved from https://www.sciencedirect.com/science/article/pii/S0009898108001782?via%3Dihub.

2. Gardella TJ, Axelrod D, Rubin D, Keutmann HT, Potts JT, Kronenberg HM, et al. Mutational analysis of the receptor-activating region of human parathyroid hormone. J Biol Chem. 1991;266:13141–6.

3. Pfister MF, Ruf I, Stange G, Ziegler U, Lederer E, Biber J, et al. Parathyroid hormone leads to the lysosomal degradation of the renal type II Na/Pi cotransporter. Proc Natl Acad Sci [Internet]. 1998;95(4):1909–14. Retrieved from http://www.pnas.org/cgi/doi/10.1073/pnas.95.4.1909.

4. Rodriguez M, Lorenzo V. Parathyroid hormone, a uremic toxin. Semin Dial. 2009;22(4):363–8.

5. Bro S, Olgaard K. Effects of excess PTH on nonclassical target organs. Am J Kidney Dis [Internet]. 1997 Nov [cited 2018 Jul 6];30(5):606–20. Retrieved from http://www.ncbi.nlm.nih.gov/pubmed/9370175.

6. Naylor SL, Sakaguchi AY, Szoka P, Hendy GN, Kronenberg HM, Rich A, et al. Human parathyroid hormone gene (PTH) is on short arm of chromosome 11. Somatic Cell Genet [Internet]. 1983 Sep [cited 2018 Jul 6];9(5):609–16. Retrieved from http://www.ncbi.nlm.nih.gov/pubmed/6353628.

7. Segre GV, Perkins AS, Witters L, Potts JT. Metabolism of parathyroid hormone by isolated rat Kupffer cells and hepatocytes. J Clin Invest. 1981;67:449–57.

8. Yamashita H, Gao P, Cantor T, Futata T, Murakami T, Uchino S, et al. Large carboxy-terminal parathyroid hormone (PTH) fragment with a relatively longer half-life than 1-84 PTH is secreted directly from the parathyroid gland in humans. Eur J Endocrinol. 2003;149(4):301–6.

9. D'AMOUR P, LAZURE C, LABELLE F. Metabolism of radioiodinated carboxy-terminal fragments of bovine parathyroid hormone in normal and anephric rats. Endocrinology [Internet]. 1985 Jul [cited 2018 Jul 6];117(1):127–34. Retrieved from http://www.ncbi.nlm.nih.gov/pubmed/4006861.

10. Cavalier E, Plebani M, Delanaye P, Souberbielle J-C. Considerations in parathyroid hormone testing. Clin Chem Lab Med [Internet]. 2015. Retrieved from http://www.degruyter.com/view/j/cclm.ahead-of-print/cclm-2015-0314/cclm-2015-0314.xml.

11. Hanon EA, Sturgeon CM, Lamb EJ. Sampling and storage conditions influencing the measurement of parathyroid hormone in blood samples: a systematic review. Clin Chem Lab Med. 2013;51(10):1925–41.

12. Schleck ML, Souberbielle JC, Delanaye P, Plebani M, Cavalier E. Parathormone stability in hemodialyzed patients and healthy subjects: comparison on non-centrifuged EDTA and serum samples with second- and third-generation assays. Clin Chem Lab Med. 2017;55(8):1152–9.

13. Vulpio C, Bossola M, Speranza D, Zuppi C, Luciani G, Di Stasio E. Influence of blood sampling site on intact parathyroid hormone concentrations in hemodialysis patients. Clin Chem [Internet]. 2010 Mar 1 [cited 2018 Jul 9];56(3):489–90. Retrieved from http://www.ncbi.nlm.nih.gov/pubmed/20190152.

14. Samuels MH, Veldhuis JD, Kramer P, Urban RJ, Bauer R, Mundy GR. Episodic secretion of parathyroid hormone in postmenopausal women: assessment by deconvolution analysis and approximate entropy. J Bone Miner Res. 1997;12(4):616–23.

15. Guillemant J, Cabrol S, Allemandou A, Peres G, Guillemant S. Vitamin D-dependent seasonal variation in growing male adolescents. Bone. 1995;17(6):513–6.

16. Nevo-Shor A, Kogan S, Joshua BZ, Bahat-Dinur A, Novack V, Fraenkel M. Seasonal changes in serum calcium, PTH and vitamin D levels in patients with primary hyperparathyroidism. Bone. 2016;89:59–63.

17. Cong E, Walker MD, Kepley A, Zhang C, McMahon DJ, Silverberg SJ. Seasonal variability in vitamin d levels no longer detectable in primary hyperparathyroidism. J Clin Endocrinol Metab [Internet]. 2015 Sep 1 [cited 2018 Jul 10];100(9):3452–9. Retrieved from https://academic.oup.com/jcem/article-lookup/doi/10.1210/JC.2015-2105.

18. Bilezikian JP, Brandi ML, Eastell R, Silverberg SJ, Udelsman R, Marcocci C, et al. Guidelines for the management of asymptomatic primary hyperparathyroidism: summary statement from the fourth international workshop. J Clin Endocrinol Metab [Internet]. 2014;99(10):3561–9. Retrieved from http://press.endocrine.org/doi/abs/10.1210/jc.2014-1413.

19. Berson SA, Yalow RS, Aurbach GD, Potts JT. Immunoassay of bovine and human parathyroid hormone. Proc Natl Acad Sci USA. 1963;49:613–7.

20. Nussbaum SR, Zahradnik RJ, Lavigne JR, Brennan GL, Nozawa-Ung K, Kim LY, et al. Highly sensitive two-site immunoradiometric assay of parathyrin, and its clinical utility in evaluating patients with hypercalcemia. Clin Chem. 1987;33(8):1364–7.

21. Quarles LD, Lobaugh B, Murphy G. Intact parathyroid hormone overestimates the presence and severity of parathyroid-mediated osseous abnormalities in uremia. J Clin Endocrinol Metab [Internet]. 1992 Jul 1 [cited 2018 Jul 11];75(1):145–50. Retrieved from https://academic.oup.com/jcem/article-lookup/doi/10.1210/jcem.75.1.1619003.

22. Wang M, Hercz G, Sherrard DJ, Maloney NA, Segre G V., Pei Y. Relationship between intact 1–84 parathyroid hormone and bone histomorphometric parameters in dialysis patients without aluminum toxicity. Am J Kidney Dis [Internet]. 1995 Nov 1 [cited 2018 Jul 11, 26(5), pp. 836–44. Retrieved from https://www.sciencedirect.com/science/article/pii/0272638695904530?via%3Dihub.

23. Lepage R, Roy L, Brossard JH, Rousseau L, Dorais C, Lazure C, et al. A non-(1-84) circulating parathyroid hormone (PTH) fragment interferes significantly with intact PTH commercial assay measurements in uremic samples. Clin Chem. 1998;44(4):805–9.

24. John, Markus R.; Goodman, William G.; Ping, Gao; Cantor, Tom; Salusky, Isidro B; Juppner H. A Novel Immunoradiometric assay detects full-length human PTH but not amino-terminally truncated fragments: implications for PTH measurements in renal failure. J Clin Endocrinol Metab. 1999;84(11):4287–90.

25. Sturgeon CM, Sprague S, Almond A, Cavalier E, Fraser WD, Algeciras-Schimnich A, et al. Perspective and priorities for improvement of parathyroid hormone (PTH) measurement—a view from the IFCC Working Group for PTH. Clin Chim Acta [Internet]. 2017;467:42–7. Retrieved from http://dx.doi.org/10.1016/j.cca.2016.10.016.

26. Kumar V, Barnidge DR, Chen LS, Twentyman JM, Cradic KW, Grebe SK, et al. Quantification of serum 1-84 parathyroid hormone in patients with hyperparathyroidism by immunocapture in situ digestion liquid chromatography-tandem mass spectrometry. Clin Chem. 2010;56(2):306–13.

27. Lopez MF, Rezai T, Sarracino DA, Prakash A, Krastins B, Athanas M, et al. Selected reaction monitoring-mass spectrometric immunoassay responsive to parathyroid hormone and related variants. Clin Chem. 2010;56(2):281–90.

28. Himmelfarb J, Stenvinkel P, Ikizler TA, Hakim RM. The elephant in uremia: oxidant stress as a unifying concept of cardiovascular disease in uremia. Kidney Int [Internet]. 2002 Nov 1 [cited 2018 Jul 12];62(5):1524–38. Retrieved from https://www.sciencedirect.com/science/article/pii/S0085253815487095?via%3Dihub.

29. Hocher B, Yin L. Why current PTH assays mislead clinical decision making in patients with secondary hyperparathyroidism. Nephron. 2017;136(2):137–42.

30. Ursem SR, Vervloet MG, Hillebrand JJG, De Jongh RT, Heijboer AC. Oxidation of PTH: in vivo feature or effect of preanalytical conditions? Clin Chem Lab Med. 2018;56(2):249–55.

31. Hocher B, Armbruster FP, Stoeva S, Reichetzeder C, Grön HJ, Lieker I, et al. Measuring parathyroid hormone (PTH) in patients with oxidative stress—do we need a fourth generation parathyroid hormone assay? PLoS One. 2012;7(7):e40242.

32. Seiler -Mussler S, Limbach AS, Emrich IE, Pickering JW, Roth HJ, Fliser D, et al. Association of nonoxidized parathyroid hormone with cardiovascular and kidney disease outcomes in chronic kidney disease. Clin J Am Soc Nephrol [Internet]. 2018;(10):CJN.06620617. Retrieved from http://cjasn.asnjournals.org/lookup/doi/10.2215/CJN.06620617.

33. Viljoen A, Singh DK, Twomey PJ, Farrington K. Analytical quality goals for parathyroid hormone based on biological variation. Clin Chem Lab Med. 2008;46(10):1438–42.

34. Ankrah-Tetteh T, Wijeratne S, Swaminathan R. Intraindividual variation in serum thyroid hormones, parathyroid hormone and insulin-like growth factor-1. Ann Clin Biochem [Internet]. 2008;45(Pt 2):167–9. Retrieved from http://acb.sagepub.com/content/45/2/167. full.

35. Moe SM, Drueke TB, Group for the KW. KDIGO clinical practice guideline for the diagnosis, evaluation, prevention and treatment of chronic kidney disease mineral and bone disorder (CKD-MBD). Kidney Int [Internet]. 2009;76(Suppl 113):S1–128. Retrieved from http://www.nature.com/ki/journal/v76/n113s/index.html.

36. Touvier M, Deschasaux M, Montourcy M, Sutton A, Charnaux N, Kesse-Guyot E, et al. Interpretation of plasma PTH concentrations according to 25OHD status, gender, age, weight status, and calcium intake: Importance of the reference values. J Clin Endocrinol Metab. 2014;99(4):1196–203.

37. Souberbielle JC, Fayol V, Sault C, Lawson-Body E, Kahan A, Cormier C. Assay-specific decision limits for two new automated parathyroid hormone and 25-hydroxyvitamin D assays. Clin Chem. 2005;51(2):395–400.

38. Cavalier E, Delanaye P, Vranken L, Bekaert A-C, Carlisi A, Chapelle J-P, et al. Interpretation of serum PTH concentrations with different kits in dialysis patients according to the KDIGO guidelines: importance of the reference (normal) values. Nephrol Dial Transplant [Internet]. 2011;27(5):1950–6. Retrieved from http://www.ncbi.nlm.nih.gov/pubmed/21940481.

Relation Between PTH and Biochemical Markers of MBD

Pablo A. Ureña-Torres, Jordi Bover and Martine Cohen-Solal

Introduction

Progressive chronic kidney disease (CKD) ineluctably leads to mineral and bone disorders (MBD). Numerous biochemical alterations observed in CKD, namely the reduced natural and active vitamin D metabolites, hypocalcemia, hyperphosphatemia, high parathyroid hormone (PTH), fibroblast growth factor 23 (FGF23), sclerostin, and low klotho, independently or in concert affect mineral and bone metabolism (CKD-MBD), and ultimately bone quality and quantity [1]. Moreover, a significant number of medications aimed to control or normalize these biological alterations often directly or indirectly impact bone metabolism, including calcium salts, intestinal phosphate binders, vitamin D compounds, calcimimetics, bisphosphonates, and other emerging therapies.

The usual circulating biomarkers of bone metabolism, either alone or combined, are poor predictors of the type of renal osteodystrophy (ROD) in CKD-MBD [2]. Thus, to establish a firm diagnosis, the qualitative and quantitative histomorphometric evaluation of a bone biopsy still remains the gold standard. The bone histomorphometric nomenclature system describes essentially five types of ROD in CKD: osteitis fibrosa or high bone turnover, adynamic bone disease,

P. A. Ureña-Torres (✉)
AURA Nord Saint Ouen, Department of Dialysis and Department of Renal Physiology, Necker Hospital, University of Paris Descartes, Paris, France
e-mail: urena.pablo@wanadoo.fr

J. Bover
Fundació Puigvert, Department of Nephrology, C./ Cartagena 340-350, 08025 Barcelona, Spain
e-mail: jbover@fundacio-puigvert.es

M. Cohen-Solal
INSERM U1132 & USPC Paris-Diderot; Department of Rheumatology; Hôpital Lariboisière, Paris, France
e-mail: martine.cohen-solal@inserm.fr

© Springer Nature Switzerland AG 2020
A. Covic et al. (eds.), *Parathyroid Glands in Chronic Kidney Disease*,
https://doi.org/10.1007/978-3-030-43769-5_7

osteomalacia, mixed lesions associating high bone turnover and osteomalacia, and osteopathies due to trace metal overload (aluminum, fluoride, strontium) [1]. This classification of CKD-MBD is mainly based on three parameters: bone formation rate (BFR) after tetracyclin double labeling, bone volume, and the amount of unmineralized osteoid surface or, in other words, the presence or not of a mineralization defect. Unfortunately, bone biopsy is still rarely indicated and performed in CKD patients, mostly because of difficulties in finding experienced teams and appropriate facilities to analyze them. Its invasive and largely perceived feeling that it is a painful procedure is an additional explanation. Therefore, considerable efforts are continuously devoted to the search of reliable noninvasive biomarkers of bone metabolism in CKD patients. These biomarkers of bone turnover in CKD-MBD would be of great importance in recognizing specific conditions, identifying patients at risk, and to guide patient tailored therapeutic intervention.

PTH is generally not considered as a biomarker of bone metabolism; however, PTH is one of the most important regulators of bone turnover and bone mineralization. Intermittent physiological doses of PTH increase bone formation and bone mass; however, extremely and constantly high or low PTH results in bone loss, increased risk of skeletal fractures and mortality [3, 4]. Regardless of the type of PTH assay, PTH values show a relatively good correlation with BFR and with most of histomorphometric parameters. However, approximately 30% of dialysis patients with normal/low BFR show PTH values between 200 and 600 pg/ml or 2–9 fold the upper limit of the reference value [5]. In spite of these findings, PTH, second and third generation assays, is the most used and useful biomarker in the diagnosis of ROD. However, one should keep in mind that PTH mostly reflects the degree of parathyroid activity and to some extent the degree of bone turnover.

Bone is composed of cells (10% osteoblasts and osteoclasts, and 90% of osteocytes) and of extracellular matrix (75% inorganic, mostly in form of hydroxyapatite, and 25% of organic proteins, mostly of type I collagen (85%) and non-collagenous compositions (15%)) [6]. Analyzing the metabolism of these proteins; collagen-related ones such as type I collagen C- and N-terminal pro-peptides (P1NP and PICP), and collagen crosslinked molecules could be a useful tool in the assessment of ROD, as well as the non-collagenous proteins such as bone-specific alkaline phosphatase (BSAP) and tartrate-resistant acid phosphatase (TRAP5b). New molecules such as fibroblast growth factor 23 (FGF23), klotho, sclerostin and Dkk1 could also emerge as interesting biomarkers of bone metabolism. In this review we will briefly update the relation of PTH with old and the most recent biomarkers of bone metabolism.

PTH and Bone Remodelling

PTH is the principal molecule controlling bone remodeling. As previously mentioned, intermittent physiological doses of PTH increases bone formation and bone mass [7, 8]; however, extremely and constantly high PTH results in bone loss and are associated with increased risk of mortality [9]. In CKD, with the decline in renal function there is alteration of the ratio between the intact and fragment forms PTH, translated by a decrease of circulating intact PTH and an increase of PTH fragments. Normal subjects have 80% of PTH fragments and 20% of intact PTH molecules, which comprises the intact PTH, N-terminal truncated PTH non 1–84 and amino-PTH [10]. On the other hand, CKD patients have 95% of PTH fragments and only 5% of the intact forms [10]. Nevertheless, whatever the type of PTH we measure, there is always a relatively good correlation between PTH, BFR and with all histological parameters as illustrated by several studies in the nineties [11, 12]. In one of these studies, which examined 96 bone biopsies from patients treated by hemodialysis or peritoneal dialysis, serum PTH levels positively and significantly correlated with BFR. It is important to note that some of these patients with normal or low BFR had serum PTH levels ranging between 200 and 600 pg/ml. Comparable results were also found in another study in 97 dialysis patients where more than one third of them had histological signs of low bone turnover while having serum PTH levels over 300 pg/ml. Altogether, these results contributed to the KDIGO guidelines and the recommendation of maintaining a PTH value between two and nine times the upper limit of normal value in dialysis patients [1]. However, although the controversies, serum PTH levels, either assessed by second or third generation assays are the most useful biomarker in the diagnosis of ROD.

PTH and Calcemia

PTH plays a vital role in maintaining calcium levels in a remarkably narrow area. PTH performs this role through its actions on the kidney, the bone and indirectly on the intestine [3, 13]. In the kidney, it stimulates calcium reabsorption in the broad ascending limb of Henle's loop and distal tubule. In bone, it stimulates bone remodeling and calcium release to the extracellular milieu. In the intestine, PTH indirectly stimulates calcium absorption via active vitamin D. In fact, it stimulates the activity of 1α-hydroxylase in the renal proximal tubule and the conversion of 25OHD to calcitriol, which directly stimulates several intestinal calcium transport proteins. Disorders of secretion of PTH synthesis and/or its mode of action on the skeleton are often associated with changes in serum calcium levels.

Serum calcium levels are maintained within a narrow range by the balance between urinary calcium excretion, intestinal calcium absorption and the amount of calcium released by the bone. Any change in serum calcium levels is detected by the parathyroid calcium sensing receptor (CaR), which adjusts PTH production [14]. Decreased serum calcium levels increase PTH, which increases renal tubular calcium reabsorption, bone resorption and calcium release. On the contrary, an increase in serum calcium levels activates the CaR, decreases PTH secretion, bone resorption, and increases urinary calcium excretion. In case of CKD, the CaR gene is normal, but its expression in parathyroid cells is reduced.

PTH acts in bone through the binding and activation of the PTH receptor type 1 (PTHR1) of osteoblasts. It stimulates cortical and trabecular bone remodeling and the release of calcium to the extracellular environment. The catabolic effect of PTH is mediated through the stimulation of RANKL (receptor activator of nuclear factor beta ligand) production and the reduction of sclerostin and osteoprotegerin (OPG) production by osteoblasts. This results in an increase in osteoclastogenesis, osteoclastic activity and bone resorption [3, 4, 15]. In case of excessive production of PTH, as in case of severe secondary hyperparathyroidism in CKD, it is possible to observe hypercalcemia, which is secondary to the excessive release of calcium from the skeleton following the PTH-induced increased bone resorption and the inability of the kidney to excrete this excessive load of bone-derived calcium (tertiary hyperparathyroidism). Paradoxically, high serum calcium levels can also be observed in case of extremely low bone turnover or adynamic bone disease because of the reduced buffer activity of the skeleton and the incapacity to uptake excessive calcium load coming either from the diet or from medications together with renal failure.

PTH and Phosphatemia

PTH was also the first hormone involved in the regulation of phosphatemia [3]. By stimulating bone resorption and calcium release, PTH also releases skeletal phosphate and may lead to hyperphosphatemia. However, PTH increases urinary excretion of phosphate due to the internalization of NPT2a and NPT2c cotransporters and the decrease of renal tubular phosphate reabsorption. For this reason, the measurement of the maximal proximal tubular phosphate transport has been used for long time, and prior to the availability of reliable PTH assays, as a marker of primary hyperparathyroidism [16]. In CKD, the phosphaturic effects of PTH are limited by the progressive loss of PTHR1 in renal cells [17]. Therefore, despite the increase in PTH and the fractional urinary phosphate excretion in CKD, the urinary excretion of daily phosphate diminishes at the late CKD stages leading to hyperphosphatemia [18]. Hyperphosphatemia decreases the expression and the sensitivity to calcium of the parathyroid CaR, making parathyroid cells less sensitive to the inhibitory action of calcium on PTH synthesis, resulting in hypersecretion of PTH [19, 20].

Bone plays an essential role in the control of phosphatemia, either by releasing phosphate during bone resorption or by storing phosphate during bone mineralization. The amount of phosphate provided by the bone depends on the degree of bone remodeling, which results from the balance between osteoblastic activity and osteoclastic activity. Bone is also responsible for the production of FGF23 by osteocytes [21]. Some examples illustrate the importance of bone in the regulation of phosphatemia, the first is that of the normalization of phosphatemia, following parathyroidectomy in cases of primary and SHPT [22]. The second is bone demineralization observed in subjects with disabling mutations of NPT2a and hypophosphatemic hyperphosphaturia [23]. In CKD, accelerated bone remodeling, as in case of SHPT and mixed osteopathy, may be responsible for hyperphosphatemia. Conversely, low bone remodeling, as in osteomalacia, adynamic osteopathy and aluminum overload, can explain as well as certain hyperphosphatemias [24].

PTH and Magnesemia

Magnesium is the second most abundant intracellular cation in the body, only a tiny amount is found in the extracellular space (2%), and less than 1% is present in the plasma compartment. Magnesium is a crucial co-factor in numerous enzymatic reactions, and it is also involved in maintaining vascular tone, cardiac rhythm, platelet activity and bone formation [25]. The kidney plays a major role in magnesium metabolism through a fine-tuning regulation within the distal convoluted segment by the TRPM5 channels. In CKD, serum magnesium levels are usually increased, and it might impact bone metabolism because of its complex interdependence with PTH. PTH production by the parathyroid glands is physiologically controlled by calcium, but magnesium, although two times lesser, can also exert similar effects activating the CaR and suppressing PTH secretion [26, 27]. The suppressing effect of Mg upon PTH occurs mainly when a moderate low serum calcium concentration is present, while this effect is blunted by normal-to-high calcium concentrations [28]. Several studies have shown a negative correlation between serum magnesium and PTH levels [29, 30]. Therefore, chronic high serum magnesium levels may lead to low serum PTH levels and might play a role in the pathogenesis of adynamic bone disease, which is associated with a higher mortality risk [31, 32]. Moreover, as magnesium is a potent inhibitor of vascular calcification, low serum magnesium levels might also be involved in the setting and progression vascular calcification in CKD.

PTH and Vitamin D

Native vitamin D, cholecalciferol (D3) and ergocalciferol (D2), are pre-hormones that play an essential role in mineral and bone homeostasis. Vitamin D stimulates intestinal absorption, mainly through its dominant active metabolite $1,25OH_2D_3$, and kidney reabsorption of calcium and phosphate. In the parathyroid gland, vitamin D suppresses PTH production. Consequently, low circulating vitamin D levels invariably result in elevated serum PTH concentrations in healthy individuals as well as in CKD patients. In clinical practice, the measurement of vitamin D2 or D3 in never performed, and that of $1,25OH_2D_3$ rarely assessed. What is usually assessed is the circulating concentration of its hydroxylated form 25OHD3, which is the standard biomarker of vitamin D status. However, this value does not reflect the concentration of its active metabolite, 1,25OH2D3, but the two metabolites show a good correlation. Several institutions including WHO, institute of medicine, K-DOQI and KDIGO have defined vitamin D deficiency as a value lower than 15 ng/ml, insufficiency between 15 and 30, sufficiency greater than 30 and intoxication over 150 ng/ml. These values have been recommended based on the following four factors: the relation between vitamin D and PTH, with intestinal calcium absorption, with its association with bone mineral density or fractures, and with its relationship with fall, walk distance and muscle strength. However, most of the times the only criteria employed is its relationship with PTH.

In the general population, serum PTH and 25OHD levels are inversely correlated as it has been also found in CKD patients (Metzger). In the French cohort NephroTest™, including more than 1,000 CKD patients, we found that 80% of patients with CKD 3–5 were vitamin D deficient (25OHD < 15 ng/ml) or insufficient (25OHD 15–13 ng/ml), only 20% had normal vitamin D status [33]. In these patients, after adjusting for renal function, age, ethnicity and ionized calcium the circulating concentration of 25OHD at which PTH starts to significantly increase was of 20 ng/ml [33, 34]. Above this value of 20 ng/ml, serum PTH levels were likely to be within normal ranges. In a different smaller Spanish study, 25(OH)D < 20 ng/ml was an independent predictor of death and progression in patients with stage 3–5 CKD, with no additional benefits when patients reached the levels at or above 30 ng/ml suggested as optimal by CKD guidelines [35].

PTH and FGF23/Klotho Axis

PTH significantly increases serum FGF23 levels in healthy subjects due to a direct stimulatory effect on osteocytes and to an indirect effect through the stimulation of 1,25OH2D3 synthesis [36]. In CKD, serum phosphate levels increase with the decline of renal function, which directly and indirectly contributes to the skeletal fragility associated with CKD-MBD, through the stimulation of PTH and FGF23 production [37]. It is also accepted that serum FGF23 levels increase in CKD patients 10 to 15 ml/min of glomerular filtration rate (GFR) earlier than PTH (break-point at 57 ml/min for FGF23 compared to 46 ml/min for PTH) [38]. In normal conditions, FGF23 inhibits PTH production and parathyroid cell proliferation through the stimulation of parathyroid CaR and VDR expression [39, 40]. However, in CKD, the hyperplastic parathyroid cells show a hyporesponsiveness to the inhibitory effect of FGF23. FGF23 fails inhibiting PTH synthesis and does not affect the parathyroid expression of CaR and VDR, partially due to a reduced klotho and FGFR1 expression [39].

Circulating levels of FGF23 have also been found to be the most important factor predicting the development of refractory SHPT in dialysis patients. Indeed, it was observed that after 2-year of follow-up, and although with comparable basal PTH values, dialysis patients with basal cFGF23 >7500 n/L were those who significantly increased their serum PTH levels and become resistant to active vitamin

D therapy [41]. Moreover, in dialysis patients with severe SHPT there is a closed correlation between serum PTH and FGF23 levels, and the reduction of PTH by surgical parathyroidectomy is followed by a significant decrease in serum FGF23 concentrations [42]. Similarly, in dialysis patients with SHPT, the proportion of patients showing a reduction of >30% in FGF23 was higher in those treated by an oral or iv calcimimetic than with a placebo [43] [44]. In addition, the oral calcimimetic-induced reductions in FGF23 were associated with lower rates of cardiovascular death and cardiovascular events [43].

FGF23 is mainly produced by osteocytes and exerts its major physiological actions in the kidney stimulating urinary phosphate excretion and inhibiting calcitriol synthesis [45]. However, it has been suggested that FGF23 could also play an important role in the regulation of bone mineralization [46]. Indeed, in the absence of FGF23, as in FGF23 knockout animals, as well as in the excess of FGF23 such as in klotho knockout animals, there is a severe bone mineralization defect [45, 46]. Likewise, high FGF23 values have been associated with reduced osteoid thickness and osteoid maturation time, in children with normal renal function and in CKD dialysis children [47]. This enigma appears to be deciphered as illustrated by a recent publication where it has been demonstrated that FGF23 modulates bone mineralization by regulating the tissue non-specific alkaline phosphatase (TNAP) specifically through the FGFR3 and independently of klotho. FGF23 inhibits TNAP and by this pathway increases extracellular concentration of pyrophosphate, reduces the amount of free inorganic phosphate, and indirectly stimulates osteopontin gene expression, a known mineralization inhibitor [48].

Bone Formation Biomarkers

PTH and Alkaline Phosphatases

As mentioned before, the cellular constituent of bone tissue is composed by 10% of osteoblasts and osteoclasts, and 90% of osteocytes [49]. These cells produce an extracellular matrix which can be divided in inorganic matrix (75%), mostly in form of hydroxyapatite and organic matrix (25%), mostly constituted of type I collagen (85%) and non-collagenous proteins (15%). Therefore, analyzing the cellular metabolism and the proteins composing the 25% of the bone matrix can be a useful tool in the assessment of ROD. Among these proteins, bone-specific alkaline phosphatase and osteocalcin are the most used biomarkers of bone formation and TRAP of bone resorption [50].

Alkaline phosphatases are membrane-bound glycoprotein enzymes favoring phosphatase ester hydrolysis, and phosphate available for mineralization. The tissue-specific alkaline phosphatases (AP) are coded by 3 genes: intestinal, placental and stem cells [51]. The tissue-non-specific alkaline phosphatases (TNALP) are coded by a single gene and they differ by a post-transcription glycosylation, which gives rise to BSAP, liver and kidney isoforms. They are cleaved by phospholipase

C and D and released to the circulation. Three AP isoforms are usually found in the circulation, 50% as BSAP, 45% of liver AP and 5% of tissue-specific AP. In addition, a recent isoform that only circulates in the serum of CKD patients has been reported [52]. They are degraded by the liver and their serum concentration is not modified by the renal function. BSAP has a molecular weight of 80 kDa and a relative long half-life of 1–5 days.

Serum BSAP levels positively correlate with PTH in dialysis patients. Moreover BSAP distinguishes better than PTH and total alkaline phosphatases normal/low bone turnover disease from high bone turnover disease in dialysis patients. BSAP equal or higher than 20 ng/ml, alone or combined with PTH of 200 pg/ml, had the highest sensitivity, specificity, and predictability values for the diagnosis of high turnover bone disease and excluded patients with normal or low turnover bone disease (Table 1) [51, 53]. In another study carried out on 137 HD patients, those with reduced distal radius BMD had a significantly higher serum BSAP levels than those without BMD reduction [54]. High serum BSAP levels have also been demonstrated to be predictive of the skeletal response to active vitamin D treatment [55] and significantly increased in the first 3 months following surgical parathyroidectomy [22]. In conclusion, there is substantial evidence suggesting that serum BSAP level alone or in combination with PTH may be a useful tool for the biochemical estimation of the degree of bone turnover in CKD.

PTH and Osteocalcin

Osteocalcin is mainly produced by osteoblasts. Its gamma-carboxylated inactive form deposited in the extracellular bone matrix, which is transformed in the active, uncarboxylated (uOC) form, after bone resorption, and released into the circulation [56]. In the circulation, 74% of the total osteocalcin circulates in its intact form, and 26% as fragments. Among them, at least 4 fragments, N-terminal, mid-region N-terminal, mid-region C-terminal and C-terminal osteocalcin [57, 58].

Table 1 Plasma bone-specific alkaline phosphatase (BSAP) and parathyroid hormone (PTH) levels in dialysis patients with high bone turnover

High bone turnover	PTH ≥ 200	Total AP ≥ 200	BSAP ≥ 20	PTH ≥ 200 BSAP ≥ 20
Sensitivity (%)	72	50	100	100
Specificity (%)	80	90	100	80
PPV (%)	92	94	84	94
NPV (%)	47	36	100	100

BSAP Bone-specific alkaline phosphatase; *PTH* Parathyroid hormone; *PPV* Positive predictive value; *NPV* Negative predictive value. BSAP equal or higher than 20 ng/ml, alone or combined with PTH of 200 pg/ml, had the highest sensitivity, specificity, and predictability values for the diagnosis of high turnover bone disease and excluded patients with normal or low turnover bone disease

Serum uOC levels are significantly and progressively lower in subjects with declining renal function compared with those of healthy individuals. They are also closely associated with the risk of subclinical atherosclerosis in CKD subjects [59]. It has been demonstrated that serum total OC levels are significantly and positively correlated with serum PTH and BSAP levels in dialysis patients. Moreover, dialysis patients with histologically proven high bone turnover have significantly higher serum OC levels than patients with normal/low bone turnover [51]. However, and in part because of the release into the circulation of multiples OC fragments during bone resorption, serum OC levels have a poor specificity (50%) in the diagnosis of low bone turnover and adynamic osteopathy [60].

PTH and P1NP

Type I collagen is produced by osteoblast cells and secreted into the extracellular space where it serves as the skeletal mineralizing matrix. Two molecules: procollagen type 1 N-terminal extension peptide (P1NP) and procollagen type 1 C-terminal extension peptide are produced by osteoblasts, released into the circulation and used as biomarkers of bone formation. However, the results of several studies showed that the utility of type 1 collagen-related molecules, either reflecting bone formation (P1NP and P1CP) or bone resorption have been inconclusive, still needing validation by larger studies [12, 51, 61]. One of the first studies measuring P1CP, the C-terminal peptide in 37 hemodialysis patients, with available bone biopsy data, did not find any difference in serum P1CP levels between patients with low or high bone turnover disease [12]. However, in another study, serum P1NP levels significantly differed between two groups of dialysis patients, being higher in those with greater annual BMD loss and the lowest in patients with the less BMD reduction [62, 63]. Similarly, the highest tertiles of P1NP were associated with the highest risk of skeletal fractures and the lowest values of BMD at the femoral neck [64]. Generally, serum PTH levels are positively correlated with P1NP in osteoporotic post-menopausal women and in dialysis patients, but confirmatory larger studies are needed [51, 62, 65].

Bone Resorption Biomarkers

PTH and TRAP5b

TRAP is a metalloenzyme with an optimal activity in acidic conditions, product of osteoclast activity. It is therefore used as a biomarker of bone resorption rate. Serum TRAP5b levels are not affected by the decline of renal function. CKD and dialysis patients show higher serum TRAP5b levels than healthy subjects [66]. The highest quartile of TRAP5b has been associated with the greatest BMD loss at the distal radius in 58 dialysis patients [67]. Similar findings have also been found in another population of 103 dialysis patients, where the high TRAP5b quartile was associated with the lowest BMD value at the second metacarpal. Interestingly, this biomarker of bone resorption was well correlated with N-terminal telopeptide of type 1 collagen (NTX), another resorption marker [68]. Finally, serum TRAP5b levels are significantly higher in dialysis patients with SHPT than in control and in patients with normal PTH. Indeed, TRAP5b correlates better than PTH with osteoclast surface, osteoclast number, BFR and mineralization apposition rate [69].

PTH and Crosslaps

Several collagen-related molecules have been used to assess the degree of bone resorption including the NTX, the C-terminal telopeptide of type I collagen (CTX) and their crosslinked molecules pyridinoline (PYD) and deoxypyridinoline (DPD). NTX are cleared by the kidney; thus, in case of CKD, serum NTX levels increase as renal clearance decreases. However, it has been evaluated in a few studies. In CKD patients treated with a bisphosphonate (residronate), in order to prevent glucocorticoid-related bone loss, it was demonstrated that serum NTX levels decreased parallel to the reduction in bone resorption index [70]. In another study in 113 dialysis patients, the highest quartiles of NTX were associated with the greatest reduction of BMD at the distal radius [71]. Serum NTX concentration was evaluated in the Bonafide study. After one year of cinacalcet treatment of dialysis patients with SHPT, serum NTX levels significantly decreased from 378 to 249 nmol/liter, following the decreased of PTH and to the BFR [72]. Considering serum CTX levels, similar to ICTP, they did not differ between dialysis patients exhibiting high and low bone turnover (33 vs. 40 ng/ml) [12]. However, the cross-linked molecule PYD (pyridinoline) was significantly higher in patients with high bone turnover compared to low bone turnover. Serum PYD levels were also very well correlated with PTH, osteoclast surfaces and number, both markers of bone resorption [12]. Interestingly, another study in Japan corroborate our findings and found a good correlation between PYD and CTX. The highest quartile of CTX was associated with the faster bone loss at the distal radius [73]. In summary, collagen derived bone biomarkers, either of formation (P1NP and P1CP) or resorption (NTX, CTX, PYD and DPD) are eliminated by the kidney and accumulated in case of CKD. Their use as diagnostic tool in CKD-MBD need further and larger studies with bone histology.

Conclusions and Perspectives

In conclusion, CKD always leads to abnormal bone turnover, volume, and mineralization. Bone biopsy still remains the gold-standard for the diagnosis of renal osteodystrophy as well as for the monitoring of any therapy impacting bone metabolism. The relation between serum concentration of PTH and biomarkers of bone metabolism is complex and not yet fully elucidated in case of patients with CKD or treated by dialysis. PTH is not always correlated with the degree of bone remodeling and in the absence of bone histology it cannot be considered as an accurate marker. Further studies, based on bone histomorphometry, are clearly needed to better understand the predictive diagnostic value of old and new, alone or combined with PTH or other biomarkers of bone metabolism in CKD-MBD.

Disclosure PAUT has received consulting fee from Amgen, Astellas, Abbvie, AstraZeneca, GSK, Hemotech, Fresenius and Vifor Pharma FMC. JB has not received consulting fees related to this work.

References

1. KDIGO. KDIGO clinical practice guideline for the diagnosis, evaluation, prevention, and treatment of Chronic Kidney Disease-Mineral and Bone Disorder (CKD-MBD). Kidney Int Suppl. 2009(113):S1–130.
2. Bover J, Urena P, Brandenburg V, et al. Adynamic bone disease: from bone to vessels in chronic kidney disease. Semin Nephrol. 2014;34(6):626–40.
3. Potts JT. Parathyroid hormone: past and present. J Endocrinol. 2005;187(3):311–25.
4. Wein MN, Kronenberg HM. Regulation of bone remodeling by parathyroid hormone. Cold Spring Harb Perspect Med. 2018;8(8).
5. Barreto FC, Barreto DV, Moyses RM, et al. K/DOQI-recommended intact PTH levels do not prevent low-turnover bone disease in hemodialysis patients. Kidney Int. 2008;73(6):771–7.
6. Baron R. Anatomy and Ultrastructure of Bone. In: Favus MJ, editor. Primer on the metabolic bone diseases and disorders of mineral metabolism. 2nd ed. New York: Raven Press, Ltd; 1993. p. 3–9.
7. Jilka RL, O'Brien CA, Ali AA, et al. Intermittent PTH stimulates periosteal bone formation by actions on post-mitotic preosteoblasts. Bone. 2009;44(2):275–86.
8. Thomas T. Intermittent parathyroid hormone therapy to increase bone formation. Joint Bone Spine. 2006;73(3):262–9.
9. Floege J, Kim J, Ireland E, et al. Serum iPTH, calcium and phosphate, and the risk of mortality in a European haemodialysis population. Nephrol Dial Transplant. 2011;26(6):1948–55.
10. Brossard J, Cloutier M, Roy L, et al. Accumulation of a non-(1-84) molecular form of parathyroid hormone (PTH) detected by intact PTH assay in renal failure: importance in the interpretation of PTH values. J Clin Endocrinol Metab. 1996;81:3923–9.
11. Qi Q, Monier-Faugere MC, Geng Z, et al. Predictive value of serum parathyroid hormone levels for bone turnover in patients on chronic maintenance dialysis. Am J Kidney Dis. 1995;26(4):622–31.
12. Urena P, Ferreira A, Kung VT, et al. Serum pyridinoline as a specific marker of collagen breakdown and bone metabolism in hemodialysis patients. J Bone Miner Res. 1995;10(6):932–9.
13. Urena P, Kong XF, Abou-Samra AB, et al. Parathyroid hormone (PTH)/PTH-related peptide receptor messenger ribonucleic acids are widely distributed in rat tissues. Endocrinology. 1993;133(2):617–23.
14. Brown EM, Gamba G, Riccardi D, et al. Cloning and characterization of an extracellular Ca(2+)-sensing receptor from bovine parathyroid. Nature. 1993;366(6455):575–80.

15. Ma YL, Cain RL, Halladay DL, et al. Catabolic effects of continuous human PTH (1–38) in vivo is associated with sustained stimulation of RANKL and inhibition of osteoprotegerin and gene-associated bone formation. Endocrinology. 2001;142(9):4047–54.
16. Bilezikian JP, Brandi ML, Eastell R, et al. Guidelines for the management of asymptomatic primary hyperparathyroidism: summary statement from the Fourth International Workshop. J Clin Endocrinol Metab. 2014;99(10):3561–9.
17. Urena P, Kubrusly M, Mannstadt M, et al. The renal PTH/PTHrP receptor is down-regulated in rats with chronic renal failure. Kidney Int. 1994;45(2):605–11.
18. Moranne O, Froissart M, Rossert J, et al. Timing of onset of CKD-related metabolic complications. J Am Soc Nephrol. 2009;20(1):164–71.
19. Geng Y, Mosyak L, Kurinov I, et al. Structural mechanism of ligand activation in human calcium-sensing receptor. Elife. 2016;5.
20. Rodriguez M, Nemeth E, Martin D. The calcium-sensing receptor: a key factor in the pathogenesis of secondary hyperparathyroidism. Am J Physiol Renal Physiol. 2005;288(2):F253–64.
21. Komaba H, Fukagawa M. FGF23: a key player in mineral and bone disorder in CKD. Nefrologia. 2009;29(5):392–6.
22. Urena P, Basile C, Grateau G, et al. Short-term effects of parathyroidectomy on plasma biochemistry in chronic uremia. Kidney Int. 1989;36(1):120–6.
23. Prie D, Beck L, Urena P, et al. Recent findings in phosphate homeostasis. Curr Opin Nephrol Hypertens. 2005;14(4):318–24.
24. Urena Torres PA, Cohen-Solal M. Not all hyperphosphataemias should be treated. Nephrol Dial Transplant. 2018.
25. Maguire ME, Cowan JA. Magnesium chemistry and biochemistry. Biometals. 2002;15:203–10
26. Vetter T, Lohse MJ. Magnesium and the parathyroid. Curr Opin Nephrol Hypertens. 2002;11(4):403–10.
27. Kawata T, Nagano N. The calcium receptor and magnesium metabolism. Clin Calcium. 2005;15(11):43–50.
28. Rodriguez-Ortiz ME, Canalejo A, Herencia C, et al. Magnesium modulates parathyroid hormone secretion and upregulates parathyroid receptor expression at moderately low calcium concentration. Nephrol Dial Transplant. 2014;29(2):282–9.
29. Navarro JF, Mora C, Jimenez A, et al. Relationship between serum magnesium and parathyroid hormone levels in hemodialysis patients. Am J Kidney Dis. 1999;34(1):43–8.
30. Navarro JF, Mora C, Macia M, et al. Serum magnesium concentration is an independent predictor of parathyroid hormone levels in peritoneal dialysis patients. Perit Dial Int. 1999;19(5):455–61.
31. Fournier A, Oprisiu R, Moriniere P, et al. Low doses of calcitriol or calcium carbonate for the prevention of hyperparathyroidism in predialysis patients? Nephrol Dial Transplant. 1996;11(7):1493–5.
32. Sakaguchi Y, Fujii N, Shoji T, et al. Magnesium modifies the cardiovascular mortality risk associated with hyperphosphatemia in patients undergoing hemodialysis: a cohort study. PLoS ONE. 2014;9(12):e116273.
33. Urena-Torres P, Metzger M, Haymann JP, et al. Association of kidney function, vitamin D deficiency, and circulating markers of mineral and bone disorders in CKD. Am J Kidney Dis. 2011;58(4):544–53.
34. Metzger M, Houillier P, Gauci C, et al. Relation between circulating levels of 25(OH) vitamin D and parathyroid hormone in chronic kidney disease: quest for a threshold. J Clin Endocrinol Metab. 2013;98(7):2922–8.
35. Molina P, Gorriz JL, Molina MD, et al. What is the optimal level of vitamin D in non-dialysis chronic kidney disease population? World J Nephrol. 2016;5(5):471–81.
36. Burnett-Bowie SM, Henao MP, Dere ME, et al. Effects of hPTH(1-34) infusion on circulating serum phosphate, 1,25-dihydroxyvitamin D, and FGF23 levels in healthy men. J Bone Miner Res. 2009;24(10):1681–5.

37. Komaba H, Fukagawa M. FGF23-parathyroid interaction: implications in chronic kidney disease. Kidney Int. 2010;77(4):292–8.
38. Gutierrez O, Isakova T, Rhee E, et al. Fibroblast growth factor-23 mitigates hyperphosphatemia but accentuates calcitriol deficiency in chronic kidney disease. J Am Soc Nephrol. 2005;16(7):2205–15.
39. Canalejo R, Canalejo A, Martinez-Moreno JM, et al. FGF23 fails to inhibit uremic parathyroid glands. J Am Soc Nephrol. 2010;21(7):1125–35.
40. Krajisnik T, Bjorklund P, Marsell R, et al. Fibroblast growth factor-23 regulates parathyroid hormone and 1alpha-hydroxylase expression in cultured bovine parathyroid cells. J Endocrinol. 2007;195(1):125–31.
41. Nakanishi S, Kazama JJ, Nii-Kono T, et al. Serum fibroblast growth factor-23 levels predict the future refractory hyperparathyroidism in dialysis patients. Kidney Int. 2005;67(3):1171–8.
42. Sato T, Tominaga Y, Ueki T, et al. Total parathyroidectomy reduces elevated circulating fibroblast growth factor 23 in advanced secondary hyperparathyroidism. Am J Kidney Dis. 2004;44(3):481–7.
43. Moe SM, Chertow GM, Parfrey PS, et al. Cinacalcet, fibroblast growth factor-23, and cardiovascular disease in hemodialysis: the Evaluation of Cinacalcet HCl Therapy to Lower Cardiovascular Events (EVOLVE) Trial. Circulation. 2015;132(1):27–39.
44. Block GA, Bushinsky DA, Cheng S, et al. Effect of etelcalcetide vs. cinacalcet on serum parathyroid hormone in patients receiving hemodialysis with secondary hyperparathyroidism: a randomized clinical trial. JAMA. 2017;317(2):156–64.
45. Shimada T, Kakitani M, Yamazaki Y, et al. Targeted ablation of Fgf23 demonstrates an essential physiological role of FGF23 in phosphate and vitamin D metabolism. J Clin Invest. 2004;113(4):561–8.
46. Shimada T, Mizutani S, Muto T, et al. Cloning and characterization of FGF23 as a causative factor of tumor-induced osteomalacia. Proc Natl Acad Sci USA. 2001;98(11):6500–5.
47. Wesseling-Perry K, Pereira RC, Wang H, et al. Relationship between plasma fibroblast growth factor-23 concentration and bone mineralization in children with renal failure on peritoneal dialysis. J Clin Endocrinol Metab. 2009;94(2):511–7.
48. Murali SK, Andrukhova O, Clinkenbeard EL, et al. Excessive osteocytic Fgf23 secretion contributes to pyrophosphate accumulation and mineralization defect in hyp mice. PLoS Biol. 2016;14(4):e1002427.
49. Bover J, Urena P, Aguilar A, et al. Alkaline phosphatases in the complex chronic kidney disease-mineral and bone disorders. Calcif Tissue Int. 2018;103(2):111–24.
50. Mazzaferro S, Tartaglione L, Rotondi S, et al. News on biomarkers in CKD-MBD. Semin Nephrol. 2014;34(6):598–611.
51. Urena P, De Vernejoul MC. Circulating biochemical markers of bone remodeling in uremic patients. Kidney Int. 1999;55(6):2141–56.
52. Haarhaus M, Fernstrom A, Magnusson M, et al. Clinical significance of bone alkaline phosphatase isoforms, including the novel B1x isoform, in mild to moderate chronic kidney disease. Nephrol Dial Transplant. 2009;24(11):3382–9.
53. Couttenye MM, D'Haese PC, VanHoof VO, et al. Bone alkaline phosphatase (BAP) compared to PTH in the diagnosis of adynamic bone disease (ABD). Nephrol Dial Transplant. 1994;9:905 (Abst.).
54. Ueda M, Inaba M, Okuno S, et al. Serum BAP as the clinically useful marker for predicting BMD reduction in diabetic hemodialysis patients with low PTH. Life Sci. 2005;77(10):1130–9.
55. Urena P, Bernard-Poenaru O, Cohen-Solal M, et al. Plasma bone-specific alkaline phosphatase changes in hemodialysis patients treated by alfacalcidol. Clin Nephrol. 2002;57(4):261–73.
56. Ferron M, McKee MD, Levine RL, et al. Intermittent injections of osteocalcin improve glucose metabolism and prevent type 2 diabetes in mice. Bone. 2012;50(2):568–75.

57. Garnero P, Grimaux M, Seguin P, et al. Characterization of immunoreactive forms of human osteocalcin generated in vivo and in vitro. J Bone Miner Res. 1994;9(2):255–64.
58. Rosenquist C, Qvist P, Bjarnason N, et al. Measurement of a more stable region of osteocalcin in serum by ELISA with two monoclonal antibodies. Clin Chem. 1995;41(10):1439–45.
59. Zhang M, Ni Z, Zhou W, et al. Undercarboxylated osteocalcin as a biomarker of subclinical atherosclerosis in non-dialysis patients with chronic kidney disease. J Biomed Sci. 2015;22:75.
60. Couttenye MM, D'Haese PC, VanHoof VO, et al. Low serum levels of alkaline phosphatase of bone origin: a good marker of adynamic bone disease in haemodialysis patients. Nephrol Dial Transplant. 1996;11:1065–72.
61. Couttenye MM, D'Haese PC, Deng J, et al. High prevalence of adynamic bone disease diagnosed by biochemical markers in a wide sample of the European CAPD population. Nephrol Dial Transplant. 1997;12:2144–50.
62. Cavalier E, Delanaye P, Collette J, et al. Evaluation of different bone markers in hemodialyzed patients. Clin Chim Acta. 2006;371(1–2):107–11.
63. Ueda M, Inaba M, Okuno S, et al. Clinical usefulness of the serum N-terminal propeptide of type I collagen as a marker of bone formation in hemodialysis patients. Am J Kidney Dis. 2002;40(4):802–9.
64. Nickolas TL, Cremers S, Zhang A, et al. Discriminants of prevalent fractures in chronic kidney disease. J Am Soc Nephrol. 2011;22(8):1560–72.
65. Dusceac R, Niculescu DA, Dobre R, et al. Chronic hemodialysis is associated with lower trabecular bone score, independent of bone mineral density: a case-control study. Arch Osteoporos. 2018;13(1):125.
66. Yamada S, Inaba M, Kurajoh M, et al. Utility of serum tartrate-resistant acid phosphatase (TRACP5b) as a bone resorption marker in patients with chronic kidney disease: independence from renal dysfunction. Clin Endocrinol (Oxf). 2008;69(2):189–96.
67. Shidara K, Inaba M, Okuno S, et al. Serum levels of TRAP5b, a new bone resorption marker unaffected by renal dysfunction, as a useful marker of cortical bone loss in hemodialysis patients. Calcif Tissue Int. 2008;82(4):278–87.
68. Hamano T, Tomida K, Mikami S, et al. Usefulness of bone resorption markers in hemodialysis patients. Bone. 2009;45(Suppl 1):S19–25.
69. Chu P, Chao TY, Lin YF, et al. Correlation between histomorphometric parameters of bone resorption and serum type 5b tartrate-resistant acid phosphatase in uremic patients on maintenance hemodialysis. Am J Kidney Dis. 2003;41(5):1052–9.
70. Fujii N, Hamano T, Mikami S, et al. Risedronate, an effective treatment for glucocorticoid-induced bone loss in CKD patients with or without concomitant active vitamin D (PRIUS-CKD). Nephrol Dial Transplant. 2007;22(6):1601–7.
71. Hamano T, Fujii N, Nagasawa Y, et al. Serum NTX is a practical marker for assessing antiresorptive therapy for glucocorticoid treated patients with chronic kidney disease. Bone. 2006;39(5):1067–72.
72. Behets GJ, Spasovski G, Sterling LR, et al. Bone histomorphometry before and after long-term treatment with cinacalcet in dialysis patients with secondary hyperparathyroidism. Kidney Int. 2015;87(4):846–56.
73. Okuno S, Inaba M, Kitatani K, et al. Serum levels of C-terminal telopeptide of type I collagen: a useful new marker of cortical bone loss in hemodialysis patients. Osteoporos Int. 2005;16(5):501–9.

Effect of PTH on the Hematologic System

Naoto Hamano, Hirotaka Komaba and Masafumi Fukagawa

Introduction

Bone consists of cells and extracellular matrices composed of an inorganic component such as calcium phosphate and an organic substance such as collagen. Bone matrix formation is mainly regulated by coordinated action of three kinds of cells, osteoblasts, osteoclasts, and osteocytes. Osteoblasts are derived from mesenchymal stem cells, regulate osteogenesis, and ultimately transform into osteocytes. Osteoclasts are formed by differentiation and fusion of bone marrow-derived monocyte/macrophage progenitor cells.

Bone marrow (BM) is composed of hematopoietic stem cells (HSCs) and marrow stromal cells. HSCs are defined as cells which possess the ability of self-renewal and of differentiation into all blood cell lineages including leukocytes, erythrocytes, and platelets (Table 1) [1]. A specific microenvironment consisting of HSCs and surrounding supportive tissues is called HSCs niche, in which crosstalk among HSCs and other numerous cells is involved in normal hematopoiesis [2]. Marrow stromal cells, also called mesenchymal stem cells, are non-hematopoietic stem cells, and can differentiate into osteoblasts, chondrocytes, adipocytes, or skeletal muscle cells.

It has been reported that PTH not only regulates bone metabolism but also affects blood cell production and function. Hyperparathyroidism (HPT) suppresses normal hematopoiesis via myelofibrosis, while PTH has been shown to have

N. Hamano · H. Komaba · M. Fukagawa (✉)
Division of Nephrology, Endocrinology and Metabolism, Tokai University School
of Medicine, 143, Shimokasuya, Isehara 2591193, Japan
e-mail: fukagawa@tokai-u.jp

N. Hamano
e-mail: nhamano@tokai.ac.jp

H. Komaba
e-mail: hkomaba@tokai-u.jp

© Springer Nature Switzerland AG 2020
A. Covic et al. (eds.), *Parathyroid Glands in Chronic Kidney Disease*,
https://doi.org/10.1007/978-3-030-43769-5_8

Table 1 Cells in bone marrow

Precursors	Mature cells
Hematopoietic stem cells	
Myeloid lineage	
BFU-C, CFU-C, Erythroblasts	Erythrocytes
Megakaryocytes	Platelets
CFU-M	Monocytes, Macrophages
CFU-G	Polymorphonuclear leukocytes
Lymphoid lineage	
Pre-pro-B, Pro-B, Pre-B	B cells
Pro-T, Pre-T	T cells
Pre-NK	NK cells
Mesenchymal stem cells	
Preosteoblasts	Osteoblasts, osteocytes
Preadipocytes	Adipocytes
Prechondrocytes	Chondrocytes
Skeletal myoblasts	Skeletal myocytes

a potential to improve survival of HSCs by acting directly or indirectly on these cells. Furthermore, recent studies focused on the interaction between osteoblasts and HSCs, revealing that HSCs niche lines selectively on the surface of the endosteum similarly to osteoblasts [3] and that PTH influences the interaction between HSCs and osteoblastic lineage. In this chapter, we summarize the pathological effects of PTH on the proliferation and viability of erythrocytes, leukocytes, and platelets, and also outline recent reports on the physiological roles of PTH in hematopoiesis.

PTH and Erythropoiesis

Immature erythroid progenitor cells in the BM are stimulated by erythropoietin (EPO), differentiate into mature erythrocytes, and are released into peripheral circulation. Normal mature erythrocytes have a lifespan of approximately 120 days [4], and old erythrocytes are destroyed in the liver and spleen. Decreased production or increased breakdown of normal erythrocytes could result in decreased hemoglobin concentrations and insufficient oxygen supply. This condition is called anemia.

End stage renal disease (ESRD) is associated with a high incidence of anemia and secondary HPT (SHPT). Renal anemia is mainly caused by an impaired production of EPO in the kidney for maintaining normal hemoglobin levels. Besides, many other factors could be involved in the pathogenesis of anemia, including iron deficiency, inflammation, bleeding, and malnutrition. In addition, several studies have suggested that SHPT may also play a role in the pathogenesis renal anemia.

Pathogenesis of Anemia Associated with Hyperparathyroidism

Myelofibrosis

Myelofibrosis is characterized by extensive fibrosis of the BM, resulting in anemia, hepatosplenomegaly, and extramedullary hematopoiesis [5]. Primary myelofibrosis is observed in patients with myeloproliferative diseases due to gene mutations in HSCs, whereas secondary myelofibrosis develops in patients suffering from solid tumors. SHPT is also known as a possible cause of such secondary myelofibrosis [6]. Recent studies investigated the pathogenetic mechanisms of myelofibrosis due to persistently high serum levels of PTH.

Lotinun et al. performed a microarray analysis on 5531 genes using mRNA extracted from the bone of rats receiving continuous administration of 1–34 PTH and found an increased expression of platelet-derived growth factor-A (PDGF-A) [7]. The investigators also confirmed that triazolopyrimidine (Trapidil), a PDGF-A inhibitor, suppresses myelofibrosis. Immunohistochemical staining revealed that PDGF-A is localized to mast cells, which suggests the interaction between myelofibrosis and mast cells. The follow-up study by Lowry et al., the same research group, showed that both the receptor tyrosine kinase inhibitor Gleevec and the phosphoinositide 3 (IP3)-kinase inhibitor wortmannin attenuated myelofiborosis in rats induced by continuous 1–34 PTH infusion. These results indicate that PDGF-A accelerates PTH-induced myelofibrosis through IP3 signaling pathways [8]. This study also demonstrated that mast cells redistribute from BM to the bone surface after PTH infusion, supporting the possibility that mature mast cells play crucial roles in the pathogenesis of myelofibrosis.

In line with these experimental studies, several clinical studies suggested that persistently high serum PTH levels are associated with myelofibrosis. Zingraff et al. performed bone biopsy before and after parathyroidectomy (PTx) in patients with SHPT and compared the extent of myelofibrosis [9]. They showed that hematocrit levels increased in patients who experienced improved myelofibrosis, suggesting that the severity of SHPT is related to the extent of myelofibrosis, that myelofibrosis is a reversible disorder, and that improvement of fibrosis might improve anemia. Rao et al. performed bone biopsy in hemodialysis patients receiving recombinant human EPO (rhEPO) and revealed that patients with EPO hyporesponsiveness had higher intact PTH levels, higher osteoclast number and eroded surface, and greater extent of myelofibrosis compared to good responders to rhEPO [10]. Taken together, these data suggest that SHPT may cause myelofibrosis and impair normal erythropoiesis, resulting in worsening of anemia and EPO hyporesponsiveness.

Inhibited Production of Erythroid Progenitor

Burst-forming unit-erythroid (BFU-E) and colony-forming unit-erythroid (CFU-E) are erythroid progenitors and are shown to express PTH/PTH-related protein receptor (PPR). This fact supports the possibility that PTH directly acts on these cells. Meytes et al. cultured BFU-E collected from human peripheral blood and showed that bovine 1–84 PTH inhibits BFU-E colony formation and that inactivation of PTH abolishes this effect [11]. However, these results were not reproduced when they used 1–34 bovine PTH, and the reasons for the discrepant results have not been elucidated so far. Taniguchi et al. found that the density of BFU-E and CFU-E in BM of dialysis patients were lower than healthy volunteers [12]. The researchers also obtained CFU-E from BM of healthy volunteers and showed that addition of uremic sera to culture medium inhibited CFU-E colony formation. This effect was more pronounced with higher PTH levels in the uremic sera. They further showed that treatment with 1–34 human PTH suppressed CFU-E colony formation in a dose-dependent manner. These results indicate that PTH suppresses proliferation of early erythroid progenitor CFU-E in vitro.

However, several subsequent studies have produced conflicting results. Dunn et al. showed that addition of 1–84 bovine PTH at concentrations 10 to 100 times normal levels failed to inhibit erythropoiesis or synthesis of heme in cultured fetal mouse liver cells [13]. Komatsuda et al. examined the effect of 1–34 human PTH (maximum concentrations of 300 ng/mL) or 1–84 human PTH (maximum concentrations of 5000 pg/mL) on CFU-E or BFU-E collected from healthy volunteers and found that neither erythropoiesis nor granulomonopoiesis were suppressed by human PTH [14]. The findings of these two studies do not support the hypothesis that PTH inhibits erythropoiesis. Thus, taken together, it remains unclear whether PTH acts on erythroid progenitor and exert inhibitory effects on erythropoiesis.

Inhibition of Erythropoietin Synthesis

EPO is mainly secreted from the kidney and plays crucial roles in differentiation of HSCs into erythroid lineage [15, 16]. EPO production is strongly related to hypoxia inducible factor (HIF) [17]. Under normoxic conditions, hydroxylation by prolyl hydroxylases (PHD) and ubiquitination by E3 ubiquitin ligase, such as von Hippel-Lindau protein, triggers proteasome-dependent degradation of HIF and thereby suppresses transcriptional activity of HIF. By contrast, under hypoxic conditions, suppression of PHD activity inhibits HIF degradation and enhances translocation of HIF into nucleus, wherein HIF forms dimers and initiates gene expression by binding at consensus sequence, hypoxia responsive element (HRE). HIF is known to regulate the expression of more than 800 genes, including EPO, vascular endothelial growth factor (VEFG), and platelet-derived growth factor beta polypeptide (PDFGB) [18]. Binding with HRE in the FOXD-1 expressing stroma-derived cells including peritubular interstitial fibroblast-like cells, renin producing cells, or vascular smooth muscle cells leads EPO secretion [19, 20].

These hypoxic reactions are impaired in CKD patients, leading to insufficient EPO secretion and renal anemia. Administration of erythropoiesis stimulating agents (ESAs) is required to compensate for relative or absolute endogenous EPO deficiency, but hemoglobin levels do not elevate sufficiently in some dialysis patients, which is called ESA hyporesponsiveness. This condition is caused by multiple factors, including iron deficiency, inflammation, malnutrition, and SHPT.

Several studies assessed the effect of PTx on endogenous EPO concentrations. One observational study of patients with primary HPT (PHPT) demonstrated that PTx did not alter the levels of endogenous EPO [21]. However, several studies of ESRD with SHPT demonstrated significant increases in circulating EPO levels after PTx [21, 22]. Thus, elevated PTH levels might contribute to decreased endogenous EPO production in ESRD patients, although it is unclear whether this is a direct effect on EPO-producing cells. Nonetheless, in a cross-sectional study of dialysis patients by Borawski et al., serum intact PTH levels were not associated with hemoglobin or circulating EPO levels [23]. Similarly, McGonigle et al. reported that there was no association between serum intact PTH levels and hematocrit in ESRD patients receiving hemodialysis or continuous ambulatory peritoneal dialysis and that PTx did not affect serum EPO concentrations or hematocrit [24]. Collectively, it remains unclear whether PTH causes decreased EPO production or ESA hyporesponsiveness in ESRD patients.

Interestingly, a recent experimental study by Wong et al. demonstrated that in UMR106.01 mature osteoblasts, human 1–34 PTH reduced the expression of HIF-1α levels and HIF signaling under normoxic conditions [25]. This result raises the hypothesis that PTH may also inhibit HIF signaling in EPO-producing cells in the kidney and thereby suppress EPO production, and further research would be needed to test this possibility.

Shortened Erythrocyte Survival

The lifetime of human erythrocytes is approximately 120 days [4]. ATP plays crucial roles in maintenance of erythrocyte morphology. Hyperosmolarity, oxidative stress, energy depletion, hyperthermia, and a wide variety of xenobiotics and endogenous substances can trigger influx of calcium into erythrocytes and thereby decrease intracellular ATP, which causes eryptosis [26–29]. In uremic patients, PTH has been considered to shorten the lifetime of erythrocytes and several studies have examined this possibility.

Bogin et al. cultured erythrocytes collected from healthy volunteers and showed that both 1–84 bovine PTH and 1–34 bovine PTH accelerated influx of calcium into erythrocytes and increased osmotic fragility of erythrocytes [30]. In another study, Akmal et al. harvested ^{51}Cr-labelled erythrocytes from 5/6 nephrectomized dogs, those with 5/6 nephrectomy and thyroparathyroidectomy, and control animals, and compared lifetime of erythrocytes among three groups in vitro [31]. While the lifetime of erythrocytes from 5/6 nephrectomized dogs was significantly shorter than control group, the dogs undergoing 5/6 nephrectomy and thyroparathyroidectomy showed comparable lifetime of erythrocytes to control animals, thus suggesting that PTH shortens the lifetime of erythrocytes in uremic animals.

Treatment for Hyperparathyroidism and Anemia

Treatment options for SHPT include vitamin D receptor activator (VDRA), calcimimetics, percutaneous ethanol injection therapy, and PTx, whereas PTx is the standard and definitive treatment of PHPT. The major purpose of lowering PTH levels in PHPT and SHPT is amelioration of disturbed bone and mineral metabolism, but several studies have suggested that PTH-lowering therapy may also improve anemia.

Parathyroidectomy

PTx is the definitive therapy for PHPT and SHPT. Several previous studies have shown that hemoglobin levels decrease transiently after PTx but then increase in the long term. A seminal early study by Zingraff et al. showed that mean hematocrit levels increased from 24.4% to 30.9% after PTx in dialysis patients with SHPT. Furthermore, they performed bone biopsy 6 to 9 months after PTx and revealed that the rise in hematocrit was more prominent among patients showing improvement of myelofibrosis [9]. Another group also reported that improvement of anemia after PTx for SHPT was more marked among patient with more severe myelofibrosis and lower hematocrit levels at baseline [32]. These data suggest that myelofibrosis associated with severe HPT contributes to anemia and that PTx could partially reverse the myelofibrosis and resultant anemia.

However, myelofibrosis is not always associated with renal anemia in ESRD patients. Mandolfo et al. performed bone biopsy in patients with severe SHPT and found that there was no association between the extent of myelofibrosis and severity of anemia [33]. Nonetheless, they found that patients receiving ESA administrations showed significant increases in hematocrit levels and reductions in the dose of ESA after PTx, indicating improved ESA responsiveness. Similarly, Coen et al. showed that hemoglobin levels increased after PTx in 45 dialysis patients with SHPT, and this increase was consistent across different surgical procedures (i.e., subtotal PTx, and total PTx with or without autotransplantation) [34]. This study included 16 patients receiving ESA and the researchers found that hemoglobin levels increased even though the mean ESA doses were decreased. Yasunaga et al. also demonstrated a rise in hemoglobin levels 1 year after PTx in patients with SHPT. Interestingly, they also found an increase in endogenous EPO levels from 22.6 ± 6.3 mU/mL to 143.8 ± 170.1 mU/mL and serum albumin levels from 3.9 ± 0.3 g/dL to 4.2 ± 0.4 g/dL after PTx, which may explain the improved anemia after surgery [35]. Finally, Trunzo et al. demonstrated that in dialysis patients with SHPT, PTx led to elevations in hemoglobin levels and reductions in the dose of rhEPO [36]. Taken together, PTx for SHPT may improve renal anemia, and this effect may be mediated not only by amelioration of myelofibrosis but also by increased renal or extra-renal production of EPO and improved nutritional status.

Several studies have also examined the effect of PTx on anemia in PHPT. Bhadada et al. reported that approximately half of PHPT patients were complicated with anemia and 75% of these anemic patients showed myelofibrosis on bone biopsy. The investigators observed an improvement of anemia after PTx among those with preexisting myelofibrosis [37]. Thus, PTx may improve anemia in patients with severe HPT, regardless of either primary or secondary.

Calcimimetics

PTH secretion is mainly regulated by the calcium-sensing receptor (CaSR) expressed in chief cells of the parathyroid gland, which senses the change of ionized calcium concentration. Calcimimetics bind to the CaSR and allosterically inhibit the secretion of PTH. Cinacalcet was clinically applied for PHPT and SHPT, whereas newly developed etelcalcetide and evocalcet can be used exclusively for uremic patients with SHPT at present [38–40]. Cinacalcet has been used clinically for a long time and has been suggested to decrease the risk of mortality and cardiovascular disease [41, 42]. In addition, several recent reports suggest an improvement of anemia after cinacalcet prescription.

A retrospective study of 40 dialysis patients demonstrated that the doses of darbepoetin significantly decreased 1 year after the initiation of cinacalcet prescription, while hemoglobin levels remained unchanged [43]. Among responders who achieved more than 30% reduction in intact PTH levels, the changes in intact PTH levels were associated with the dose reduction of darbepoetin. Tanaka et al. performed a secondary analysis of a 3-year, multicenter, prospective cohort study on 3,201 dialysis patients with SHPT to assess whether cinacalcet use is associated with improvement of anemia. The investigators showed that cinacalcet was associated with 1.1-fold increase in the odds of achieving the target hemoglobin levels after adjustment with potential confoundings [44]. These studies suggest that cinacalcet can increase the response to ESA and thereby improve renal anemia.

Vitamin D Receptor Activator and Nutritional Vitamin D

The vitamin D receptors are expressed in chief cells of the parathyroid gland and play a role in the regulation of PTH secretion. VDRA administration and supplementation of nutritional vitamin D are thus therapeutic options for SHPT especially among patients with vitamin D deficiency. Several studies have examined whether the use of VDRA or nutritional vitamin D is associated with improvement of anemia or ESA hyporesponsiveness in dialysis patients.

Albitar et al. demostrated that in dialysis patients with SHPT, administration of alfacalcidol led to elevations in hemoglobin concentrations and reticulocyte count together with reductions in intact PTH levels [45]. Another study showed that dialysis patients receiving intravenous calcitriol showed increased hemoglobin levels along with decreased PTH levels regardless of ESA use [46]. Of note, the association of calcitriol administration with increased hemoglobin levels was found only in patients who achieved significant suppression of PTH levels. Thus, it is suggested that the improvement of anemia after VDRA administration is mediated through the reduction in PTH levels.

As for vitamin D status, it is reported that vitamin D insufficiency, defined as serum levels of 25-hydroxyvitamin D (25(OH)D) lower than 30 ng/mL, is present in more than half of dialysis patients [47]. Vitamin D deficiency has been shown to be associated with anemia [48], and several studies have examined whether supplementation of nutritional vitamin D improves ESA hyporesponsiveness.

In a small randomized study by Rianthavorn et al. comparing ergocalciferol and placebo in children with CKD and vitamin D deficiency, the ergocalciferol group showed a significant improvement of ESA hyporesponsiveness without changes in PTH levels [49]. Miskulin et al. performed a double-blind, placebo-controlled, randomized clinical trial to examine the effect of ergocalciferol on ESA responsiveness [50]. The primary outcome was the change in rhEPO dose over 6 months. The study population included 276 dialysis patients with vitamin D insufficiency, and 80% or more were concomitantly treated with VDRAs. The researchers demonstrated that intact PTH levels were comparable between ergocalciferol and placebo arms and there were no significant changes in rhEPO doses in both arms. The lack of response in intact PTH levels to ergocalciferol is consistent with the results of another randomized, placebo-controlled study showing that cholecalciferol supplementation decreased intact PTH levels in non-hemodialysis patients but not in hemodialysis patients [51]. Therefore, nutritional vitamin D supplementation has little or no effect on intact PTH levels in ESRD patients, which may explain the lack of improvement of anemia in this population.

Taken together, VDRA may improve anemia or ESA hyporesponsiveness by decreasing PTH levels, but the effect of nutritional vitamin D is much less marked in ESRD patients. The expression of vitamin D receptor is detectable in non-classical target organs including immune system (T and B cells, macrophages, and monocytes), reproductive system (uterus, testis, ovary, prostate, placenta, and mammary glands), endocrine system (pancreas, pituitary, thyroid, and adrenal cortex), muscles, brain, skin, and liver, suggesting the pleiotropic effects of vitamin D or VDRA [52]. Furthermore, a recent study demonstrated the presence of vitamin D receptor in HSCs [53]. These data support the possibility of the direct effect of vitamin D or VDRA on hematopoiesis. However, current clinical evidence in ESRD patients does not support this possibility and suggest that vitamin D or VDRA could provide improvement of anemia only when PTH levels were lowered.

Stimulatory Action of PTH for Hematopoiesis

Osteoblasts are bone-forming cells derived from mesenchymal stem cells. These cells line the endosteal surfaces and regulate calcification by producing collagen, non-collagenous protein such as osteocalcin and osteopontin, and proteoglycan such as decorin. The PPR that expresses in osteoblasts is an important mediator of bone formation and bone resorption, which is evidenced by the fact that overexpression of constitutively active PPR in transgenic mice leads to increase of both osteoblasts and osteoclasts in trabecular bone [54].

Importantly, HSCs are not distributed randomly in the BM but are more abundant near endosteal surfaces [55], and the interaction between HSCs and osteoblasts has been investigated. G-CSF and hepatocyte growth factor secreted from osteoblasts have been shown to play an important role in differentiation of HSCs [3, 56]. Furthermore, recent studies revealed that Jagged1/Notch signaling is involved in the interaction of osteoblasts and HSCs, and that PTH affects the interaction.

Notch is a transmembrane receptor that plays an essential role in cell differentiation and function and regulates the cell-fate specification by binding of its ligand Jagged1. Osteoblasts are one of the cells that produces Jagged1 whose expression is increased by PTH [57, 58]. Jagged1 produced by osteoblasts not only regulates cell-fate determination by activating Notch 1 in an autocrine manner but also affects HSCs proliferation by activating Notch 1 in these cells (Fig. 1) [57, 58]. Furthermore, in mices undergoing allogenic BM transplantation, 1–34 rat PTH administration, given 5 times a week for four weeks followed by lethal irradiation, was beneficial for survival of grafted HSCs [57].

In addition to the Jagged1/Notch signaling, cadherin-11 is also shown to be involved in the interaction of osteoblasts and HSCs regulated by PTH (Fig. 1). Cadherin-11 is an adhesion molecule that is selectively expressed by stromal cell-derived cells, especially fibroblasts, and is thought to be one of the important inflammatory mediators [59]. Yao et al. isolated and expanded marrow stromal cells obtained from healthy volunteers and performed coculture of these cells and isolated CD34$^+$ HSCs to investigate the effect of PTH on proliferation of CD34$^+$ HSCs [60]. The ability of culture-expanded human marrow stromal cells to expand cocultured CD34$^+$ HSCs was enhanced when cocultured with PTH, but their ability was totally eliminated when cocultured with Transwell system, suggesting that direct interaction via adhesion molecules between HSCs and marrow stromal cells are necessary for the enhancement. The researchers also demonstrated that PTH increased the expression of cadherin-11 in marrow stromal cells and that depletion of cadherin-11 expression in marrow stromal cells by small interfering RNA abolished the enhancement of HSC expansion by PTH-treated marrow stromal cells. This study suggests that cadherin-11 is an important molecule for the adhesion of marrow stromal cells to HSCs and that PTH supports proliferation of

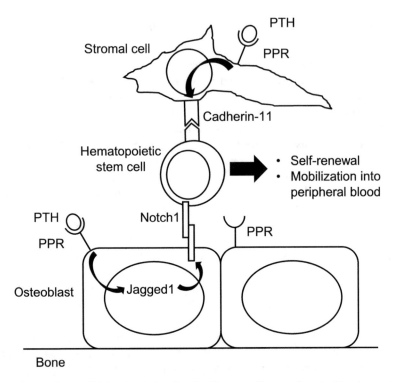

Fig. 1 Schematic of PTH-involved signaling leading to self-renewal and efflux into peripheral circulation of HSCs. HSC, hematopoietic stem cell; PTH, parathyroid hormone; PPR, PTH/PTH-related protein receptor 1

HSCs through increased expressions of cadherin-11. Furthermore, they assessed the effect of 1–34 human PTH treatment following allogenic BM transplant in lethally irradiated mice and demonstrated that PTH administration increased the expression of cadherin-11 on marrow stromal cells and improved survival rate of the mice. Collectively, these experiment data support the possibility that PTH promotes the proliferation of HSCs.

Recent studies also suggested that PTH accelerates mobilization of HSCs into peripheral circulation. One clinical study of PHPT patients showed that the HSC count in peripheral blood was significantly higher in PHPT patients than healthy volunteers and that PTx lead to reductions in the peripheral HSCs [61]. In this study population, the levels of cytokines such as vascular endothelial growth factor, which enhance mobilization of BM cells into peripheral blood, were comparable to those of healthy volunteers, suggesting that the effect of PTH to promote HSC mobilization was independent of these cytokines. Another study by Yu et al. evaluated the effect of teriparatide (1–34 human PTH) for up to 24 months on peripheral HSCs and other hematologic markers in patients with postmenopausal osteoporosis [62]. Only HSC count was significantly increased as early as

3 months, while the number of leukocytes, T cells, B cells, erythrocytes, and platelets did not change significantly throughout the study period. Thus, teriparatide may enhance the mobilization of HSCs into peripheral blood, although the mechanism remains largely unknown. The mobilization of HSCs into peripheral blood is known to play a role in cancer cell growth and post-infarction cardiac remodeling but is also suggested to support autologous stem cell collection.

The putative effects of PTH to increase HSCs and enhance their mobilization into peripheral circulation raise the possibility that PTH may support the engraftment after BM transplantation with a complete recovery of donor-derived hematopoiesis in leukocytes, erythrocytes, and thrombocytes. Based on these possibilities, accumulating studies have investigated the effect of PTH pretreatment on hematologic systems after BM transplantation. Ballen et al. performed phase I trial to assess the safety and efficacy of teriparatide administration for mobilization of HSCs into peripheral blood. A total of 20 patients who had 1 or 2 unsuccessful peripheral blood stem cell collections received escalating doses of 40 to 100 μg teriparatide for 14 days and 10 μg/kg filgrastim, a recombinant G-CSF agent, after myeloablative therapy [63]. Teriparatide administration was well-tolerated and successfully mobilized HSCs into peripheral blood in 40% and 47% of patients who failed 1 and 2 prior mobilization attempts, respectively. The success rate of achieving engraftment increases as more HSCs are harvested from peripheral blood. These data suggest that teriparatide is a promising agent for supporting hematopoiesis in BM transplantation.

It is known that the number of HSCs collected from umbilical cord blood (UCB) is limited, and even with the use of 2 UCB units, engraftment and immune reconstitution are often slow, leading to an elevated risk of infection and second malignancy [64, 65]. Thus, several clinical trials have been performed in an attempt to achieve early engraftment with the use of HSCs of UCB. However, previous studies have shown that ex vivo expansion of HSCs harvested from UCB did not the improve the survival of these cells after transfer to recipients [66, 67]. On the basis of accumulating evidence that PTH supports hematopoiesis and the results of the phase I trial showing that PTH pretreatment successfully mobilized HSCs into peripheral blood, phase II trial was conducted to examine the efficacy of PTH pretreatment for UCB transplantation [68]. This trial assessed whether 100 μg/day subcutaneous teriparatide administrations after a myeloablative or a reduced-intensity double UCB transplantation improves the rate of engraftment in patients indicated for UCB transplantation. All 13 patients achieved engraftment of neutrophil and platelet, but 4 patients died before day 100 due to transplant-associated complications, which led to early study closure although these deaths were not considered to be caused by teriparatide-related adverse effects. The researchers concluded that there was no evidence that PTH influenced blood count recovery. Although this study does not preclude the possibility that PTH supports engraftment after HSC transplantation, no additional trials have been performed until now and it remains unclear whether systemic administration of teriparatide after HSC transplantation is clinically beneficial.

Because teriparatide strongly induces bone formation, many clinical trials have assessed the efficacy of intermittent administration of teriparatide for postmenopausal osteoporosis. When we look into these results more closely, hematology-associated side effects were rarely reported; we found leukocytosis just in one study conducted in Japan, but the incidence rate was less than 1% [62, 69, 70]. These results suggest that the impact of teriparatide administration on mature blood cells in peripheral circulation is limited at least in postmenopausal women with osteoporosis.

Collectively, PTH administration may augment the production of HSCs and exert favorable effects on survival of HSCs. Moreover, teriparatide could induce mobilization of HSCs into peripheral blood. However, the effect of teriparatide on hematologic status in humans has not been well documented and the reason for the discrepant findings remains unknown. Further studies are needed to assess whether PTH administration increases proliferation of HSCs after transplantation and could be a novel strategy to support engraftment in this setting.

PTH and Immunity

In mammals, the immune system comprises two branches; innate immunity and acquired immunity. Both humoral and cellular factors are considered important in the immunity process. Humoral factors of innate immunity include inflammation and complement, and cellular factors include neutrophils, eosinophils, basophils, mast cells, macrophages, NK cells, and dendritic cells. As for acquired immunity, B cells engage in humoral immunity and T cells in cellular immunity.

ESRD patients are known to be immune-compromised, and it is reported that the annual mortality rate due to infectious diseases is 100 times or higher in dialysis patients than the general population [71]. Higher age, diabetes mellitus, lower albumin levels, catheter insertion, reuse of dialyzer, hyperphosphatemia, and elevated alkaline phosphatase (ALP) levels have been shown to be associated with higher infection-related mortality risk [72–74]. In addition, higher PTH levels are also shown to be associated with infectious death in dialysis patients [75]. Basic researches have shown that PTH adversely affects the function of leukocytes, which suggests that HPT has a negative impact on human immunity.

PTH and Polymorphonuclear Leukocytes

Innate immunity is the first line of defense against the invasion of foreign body or microbes into the body, wherein neutrophils, eosinophils, and basophils play essential roles. Several studies compared the function of polymorphonuclear leukocytes (PMNLs) in dialysis patients to that in healthy volunteers to estimate the effect of PTH on immune-related cell function. Massry et al. showed that elastase release from PMNLs was significantly decreased in dialysis patients [76]. Doherty et al. demonstrated that the migration of PMNLs was decreased in dialysis patients, particularly in those with higher PTH levels [77]. The same group also reported that patients with SHPT had higher resting levels of calcium and lower ATP contents in the cytosol of PMNLs. They also showed that phagocytic function was suppressed in these patients and this suppression was recovered by the calcium channel blocker verapamil [78–80]. These results raised the possibility that PTH disturbs phagocytosis or random migration of PMNLs, which could lead to impaired innate immunity. However, it should be stressed that the above studies compared PMNLs collected from patients with SHPT to those from healthy volunteers, which cannot dissociate the effect of PTH from that of other uremic toxins and thus cannot confirm the effect of PTH on the immune system. Future studies should compare the function of PMNLs among dialysis patients with different PTH levels.

PTH and Macrophages

Macrophages are mononuclear cells of the myeloid lineage and are originally derived from HSCs. Macrophages are not only circulating in the peripheral blood but also reside as Kupffer cells in the liver, as Langerhans cells in the lung, and as microglia in the brain. For decades, osteoclasts have been considered as macrophages that reside in bone. However, osteoclasts do not express F4/80 antigen that can be detected in almost all the other local resident macrophages. Indeed, osteoclasts were not diminished in macrophage Fas-induced apoptosis (MAFIA) transgenic mice, which allow for conditional depletion of macrophages, indicating that osteoclasts originate from myeloid progenitor that are different from other resident macrophages [81, 82]. Of note, several researchers confirmed the existence of F4/80 positive cells in BM that are distinct from osteoclasts [83]. These cells are called osteal macrophages and have been shown to control the function of osteoblasts in the vicinity of those cells.

Chang et al. demonstrated that the MAFIA transgenic mice do not have mature osteoblasts and show alterations in bone mineralization [83]. The researchers further performed coculture of osteoblasts and osteal macrophages and demonstrated that osteoblasts induce calcification only when cocultured with osteal macrophages, suggesting that osteal macrophages play an important role in mineralization induced by osteoblasts. Cho et al. also showed that intermittent PTH injection to mice increased osteal macrophages in endosteum and periosteum areas [81]. They also demonstrated that the MAFIA mice showed decreased cortical and trabecular bone volume and that PTH injection did not stimulate bone formation. These data suggest that osteal macrophages play a crucial role in the PTH-induced acceleration of bone formation.

Taken together, it can be considered that osteal macrophages play a key role in the regulation of bone metabolisms through crosstalk with osteoblasts. Much remains to be known about the nature and the mechanism of osteoclast differentiation, and further researches are needed to determine the role of PTH in this process.

PTH and B Cells

B cells are central mediators in humoral immunity and recognize bacteria and viruses and assist in the immune process through synthesis and release of antibodies. Human and bovine lymphocytes are known to express the PPR, and PTH has been shown to affect the function of B cells by activating adenylate cyclase [84].

Alexiewicz et al. obtained peripheral blood from healthy volunteers and dialysis patients and assessed the effects of PTH on the functions of isolated B cells [85]. The researchers confirmed the expression of the PPR in B cells and demonstrated that PTH acts on B cells directly and inhibits their differentiation by increasing intracellular production of cAMP. Gaciong et al. showed that bovine 1–84 PTH and synthetic bovine 1–34 PTH inhibited *Staphylococcus aureus*-stimulated production of immunoglobulin by cultured monocytes that were obtained either from dialysis patients or normal subjects [86]. They also showed that in 5/6 nephrectomized rats, PTx led to reductions in the amount of anti-*Staphylococcus aureus* antibody [87]. These findings suggest that PTH inhibits the differentiation and function of B cells at least in the setting of SHPT.

Kotzmann et al. examined 12 PHPT patients before and 6 months after PTx and 9 sex- and age-matched control subjects to determine the impact of PTH on serum immunoglobulin levels and immunophenotype of peripheral blood lymphocytes [88]. They found that immunoglobulin levels in PHPT patients did not change after PTx and were comparable to control subjects. Similarly, levels of T lymphocytes (CD3), B lymphocytes (CD19), NK cells (CD16/56) and monocytes (CD16) also did not change after PTx. Thus, the impact of high PTH on immune systems is relatively small in PHPT patients compared to that in SHPT patients.

The effect of PTH on B cells has not been explored in previous clinical trials of teriparatide for osteoporotic patients. It remains thus unknown whether intermittent administration of 1–34 PTH affects B cell differentiation and function.

PTH and T Cells

T cells are another class of lymphocytes and play an important role in immunity. T cells undergo an instructional process of positive and negative selection in the thymus. Mature T cells can be divided into different subgroups, namely CD4$^+$ T cells which produce cytokines and interact with B cells, CD8+ T cells which exert cytotoxic effects on infected cells or cancer cells, and regulatory T cells which are considered to protect against autoimmune diseases [89]. In experimental studies, researchers often use phytohemagglutinin (PHA), which is one of the plant lectins and stimulates T cell blastoid transformation, differentiation, and proliferation through T cell receptors. It is well accepted that the extent of PHA-induced lymphocyte proliferation is an indicator of T cell-mediated immunity.

Interleukin 2 (IL2) produced by T cells plays crucial roles in proliferation and differentiation of T and B lymphocytes. The expression of IL2 depends on cytosolic calcium concentrations of T cells. PTH induces influx of calcium into variety of cells and, for that reason, may affect the synthesis of IL2 by T cells. Klinger et al. isolated lymphocytes from healthy subjects and examined whether addition of 1–34 bovine PTH or 1–84 bovine PTH affects IL2 production and PHA-induced T cell proliferation [90]. The investigators found that both 1–34 PTH and 1–84 PTH accelerated PHA-induced T cell proliferation dose-dependently, while inactivated 1–84 PTH did not produce a similar effect. Of note, PTH is known to increase intracellular cAMP through the PPR, but in this study, forskolin, a stimulator of intracellular cAMP levels, did not induce T cell proliferation, suggesting that PTH stimulates T cell proliferation through the cAMP-independent pathways. They also demonstrated that PHA-induced IL2 production was enhanced with 1–84 PTH treatment. These results indicate that PTH stimulates both T cell proliferation and IL2 production.

However, these experimental results were not confirmed in clinical studies. Tzanno-Martins et al. examined T cell function in patients with severe SHPT (average intact PTH 1,425 ± 623 pg/mL) who underwent PTx [91]. The investigators showed that lymphoproliferative response to PHA was significantly increased 4 months after PTx, but there were no significant changes in IL2.

Kotzmann et al. examined PHPT patients and showed increased proportion of CD4+ T cells and decreased proportion of CD8+ T cells compared to normal subjects [88]. However, PTx for these patients did not change the number of CD4+ T cells and CD8+ T cells, suggesting the impact of PTH on CD4/CD8 ratio was limited. Taken together, it remains unclear whether PTH affects T cell function and cellular immunity, and additional research is needed to confirm this interaction.

PTH and Bone Cell-Immune Cell Crosstalk

HSCs form specific microenvironment in BM, called as niche, and crosstalk between HSCs and adjacent cells is quite important for differentiation and proliferation of HSCs. Immune cells are derived from HSCs and released into peripheral circulation after differentiation from HSCs. Increasing evidence suggests that PTH plays an important role in crosstalk between HSCs and adjacent cells for differentiation of immune-related cells, especially B cells and T cells.

Tokoyoda et al. first demonstrated the importance of BM niche in B cell development by showing that early B cell progenitors directly contact marrow stromal cells expressing C-X-C motif chemokine 12 (CXCL12) and IL-7 [92]. Several studies subsequently revealed that marrow stromal cells in the BM niche are important for B cell differentiation and that osteoblast lineage supports hematopoiesis. Furthermore, the PPR signaling, which is essential for differentiation of osteoblast lineage, has been shown to accelerate differentiation and maturation of lymphocytes.

Zhu et al. demonstrated that B cell differentiation require their attachment to osteoblasts, which is mediated via osteoblast-expressed vascular cell adhesion molecule 1 (VCAM1), stromal-cell-derived factor 1 (SDF1), and IL-7 signalling induced by PTH [93]. The researchers also revealed that addition of c-Kit ligand, IL-6, and IL-3 produced by nonosteoblastic stromal cells induce myelopoiesis. Furthermore, transgenic mice with selective elimination of osteoblasts showed severely depleted pre-pro-B and pro-B cells from BM. These results reinforced the importance of osteoblasts in B cell commitment and maturation. Based on the fact that the G protein α subunit, Gsα, is one of the downstream mediators of PPR signaling, Wu et al. generated mice with osteoblast lineage-specific deletion of Gsα using Osx1-Cre to examine the effect of Gsα on B cell differentiation and explore chemokines involved in this process [94]. As expected, the osteoblast-specific Gsα-KO mice showed marked reductions in B cell precursors both in the BM and in the peripheral blood. These mice also showed decreased serum IL-7 levels, and subcutaneous injection of IL-7 partially restored the number of pro-B cells and pre-B cells. These data suggest that Gsα-dependent signaling pathways in osteoblast lineage cells regulate differentiation and proliferation of B cells, at least partially in an IL-7-dependent manner.

Panaroni et al. examined the differences in B lymphopoiesis between mice with Osx1-Cre-mediated deletion of PPR in osteoblast lineage cells, those with osteocalcin-Cre-mediated deletion in mature osteoblasts, and those with Dmp1-Cre-mediated deletion in osteocytes [95]. Compared to control mice, the transgenic mice with PPR deletion in osteoblast lineage cells showed a decreased number of B cells, comparable expression of CXCL12, and reduced expression of IL-7 in BM. By contrast, B cell precursors were increased in BM in mice with either mature osteoblast- or osteocyte-specific deletion of the PPR. These results suggest that PTH acts on immature osteoblast lineage cells and stimulates IL-7 production, which in turn induces differentiation of B cell precursors, but such effects do not occur in more mature osteoblasts or osteocytes. Collectively, it can be concluded that direct contact with osteoblast lineage cells in BM niche is important for B cell differentiation and proliferation, and this effect is mediated through PTH-induced IL-7 production by osteoblast lineage cells.

While studies have shown the roles of osteoblast lineage cells in B cell differentiation and proliferation, T cells have been shown to play a role in differentiation and proliferation of osteoblast lineage cells.

Gao et al. investigated the effects of continuous injection of 1–34 human PTH on bone metabolism using mice lacking T cells generated by injection of anti-CD4/CD8 antibodies [96]. Bone histomorphometry revealed that two weeks of PTH injection increased the number of osteoclasts and induced bone absorption in control mice, but not in T cell-depleted mice. The investigators further demonstrated that PTH treatment failed to increase osteoclast formation in BM derived from T cell-depleted mice, whereas the addition of CD4+ or CD8+ cells to T cell-depleted BM dose dependently increased the osteoclastogenic activity of PTH, suggesting that both CD4+ or CD8+ cells could promote osteoclast formation induced by PTH. The researchers also demonstrated that deletion of T cell-expressed CD40 ligand blunts the bone catabolic activity of PTH by decreasing bone marrow stromal cell number, the RANKL/OPG ratio, and osteoclastogenic activity. These data indicate that T cells play an essential role in increased bone resorption associated with HPT by regulating stromal cell proliferation and function through CD40L.

T cells play important roles not only in bone resorption but also in bone formation. Terauchi et al. intermittently administered 1–34 human PTH to T cell deficient mice and control mice and demonstrated that T cell null mice showed attenuation of bone formation compared to control mice [97]. The researchers also revealed that PTH increases the production of Wnt10b by CD8+ T cells in BM and thereby induces these lymphocytes to activate canonical Wnt signaling in preosteoblasts. Furthermore, intermittent PTH administration decreased apoptosis of preosteoblasts, which was less evident in T cell null mice compared to control mice. These effects could explain the decreased differentiation and proliferation of osteoblasts and reduced bone formation in the T cell null mice. These studies indicate that PTH and T cells play important roles in the differentiation from osteoblastic progenitors to mature osteoblast lineage cells. The close interaction between bone cells and immune cells in BM suggests that a full understanding of this crosstalk provide novel pharmacological targets for osteoporosis and other bone diseases.

PTH and Hemostasis

Platelets and coagulation factors are two major players in hemostasis. Primary hemostasis in the setting of bleeding due to vascular injury is achieved by contraction of blood vessels and aggregation of platelets. Arachidonic acid (AA) and adenosine diphosphate (ADP) are engaged in platelet aggregation. Circulating coagulation factors are inactive under normal circumstances, but could be sequentially activated in secondary hemostasis that occurs simultaneously with the primary hemostasis.

Thrombosis is a pathological process in which the hemostatic system is excessively activated and causes the development of platelet-aggregates that prevent normal blood circulation. This process contributes to the development of cardiovascular diseases (CVD), which is the major cause of death in ESRD patients. Many observational studies have shown associations between high PTH and elevated risk of CVD in predialysis and dialysis patients (see Chap. 9). Vascular calcification and endothelial dysfunction have been shown to mediate this association, and recent studies also suggest the involvement of platelet aggregation and coagulation in this process.

PTH and Platelets

Several clinical and experimental data suggest that PTH affects both the number and function of platelets. In one case report of a patient with PHPT, PTx led to improvement of anemia and thrombocytopenia along with improved myelofibrosis [98]. As such, the association between high PTH and myelofibrosis has been well documented, and it can be argued that elevated PTH may decrease the number of platelets through the development of myelofibrosis and thereby cause abnormal bleeding.

As for the association between PTH and the function of platelet, Ortega et al. confirmed that platelets express the PPR and showed that 1–36 PTHrP induces platelet aggregation by increasing the intracellular calcium concentration via MAP kinase pathway [99]. Because PTHrP and PTH share the same receptor (PPR), similar phenomenon can be expected with PTH. Verdoia et al. collected peripheral blood from 362 patients who received dual antiplatelet therapy of aspirin plus ADP antagonist (clopidogrel or ticagrelor) for acute coronary syndrome or after percutaneous coronary intervention for stable CVD, and examined AA-mediated and ADP-mediated platelet aggregation by measuring high residual-on-treatment platelet reactivity (HRPR) [100]. The researchers found that high intact PTH levels were associated with increased ADP-mediated platelet aggregation in patients with clopidogrel but not those with ticagrelor. These findings may suggest that PTH modulates the effect of ADP antagonist, but the reason for the discrepancy between clopidogrel and ticagrelor is unknown. Collectively, PTH may induce abnormal platelet aggregation, but it remains unclear whether the effect of PTH on platelet aggregation mediates the association between HPT and CVD.

PTH and Coagulopathy

While excessive platelet aggregation can cause thrombosis in artery, activation of coagulation factors can lead to venous thrombosis, such as deep vein thrombosis and pulmonary thromboembolism. Hepatocytes, which produce coagulation factors, are known to express the PPR [101], raising the possibility that PTH affects the production of coagulation factors.

Several case reports have demonstrated the occurrence of venous thrombus in PHPT patients. Pringle et al. reported two cases of renal venous thrombosis associated with PHPT [102]. Manosroi et al. reported a case of subclavian venous thrombosis and pulmonary embolisms associated with parathyroid carcinoma [103]. However, it should be mentioned that hypercalcemia associated with PHPT can cause renal diabetes insipidus, and the resultant hemoconcentration might have led to thrombus formation in these patients. Thus, it remains unknown whether PTH directly affects coagulation or thrombus formation.

Several researchers examined the association between PTH levels and coagulation factors in patients with PHPT or SHPT. Erem et al. showed that PHPT patients had higher tissue plasminogen activator (t-PA) and plasminogen activator inhibitor (PAI)-1 and lower tissue factor pathway inhibitor (TFPI) compared to healthy volunteer, suggesting a hypercoagulability and hypofibrinolytic state in these patients [104]. However, another research group performed a case-control study and revealed that PTx did not change plasma coagulation factors such as PAI-1 in PHPT patients [105]. Another cohort study demonstrated that in patients with HPT secondary to vitamin D deficiency, vitamin D supplementation did not change coagulation factors, such as prothrombin time, activated partial thromboplastin time, factors VII, VIII, and X, even though these patients showed a significant reduction in PTH levels [106]. Thus, it is unclear whether PTH affects the production of coagulation factors.

Conclusion

Over the past decades, many studies have focused on the adverse effects of PTH, which can cause myelofibrosis, anemia, and immunosuppression particularly in patients with PHPT and SHPT. However, recent investigations have also uncovered that PTH mediates crosstalk between HSCs and marrow stromal cells including osteoblasts, osteoclasts, and osteal macrophages, and represents an important player in differentiation and proliferation of these cells. Despite the accumulation of basic research showing the potential abilities of PTH to support hematopoiesis, there are only a few evidences supporting the clinical benefit of PTH in terms of hematopoiesis. Future research should examine whether PTH administration supports hematopoiesis and improves the outcome of BM transplantation.

References

1. Metcalf D. Concise review: hematopoietic stem cells and tissue stem cells: current concepts and unanswered questions. Stem Cells. 2007;25(10):2390–5.
2. Birbrair A, Frenette PS. Niche heterogeneity in the bone marrow. Ann N Y Acad Sci. 2016;1370(1):82–96.

3. Taichman RS, Reilly MJ, Emerson SG. Human osteoblasts support human hematopoietic progenitor cells in vitro bone marrow cultures. Blood. 1996;87(2):518–24.
4. Dagg JH, Horton PW, Orr JS, Shimmins J. A direct method of determining red cell lifespan using radioiron: an application of the occupancy principle. Br J Haematol. 1972;22(1):9–19.
5. Tefferi A. Myelofibrosis with myeloid metaplasia. N Engl J Med. 2000;342(17):1255–65.
6. Albright F, Aub JC, Bauer W. Hyperparathyroidism: A common and polymorphic condition as illustrated by seventeen proved cases from one clinic. JAMA. 1934;102(16):1276–87.
7. Lotinun S, Sibonga JD, Turner RT. Triazolopyrimidine (trapidil), a platelet-derived growth factor antagonist, inhibits parathyroid bone disease in an animal model for chronic hyperparathyroidism. Endocrinology. 2003;144(5):2000–7.
8. Lowry MB, Lotinun S, Leontovich AA, Zhang M, Maran A, Shogren KL, et al. Osteitis fibrosa is mediated by Platelet-Derived Growth Factor-A via a phosphoinositide 3-kinase-dependent signaling pathway in a rat model for chronic hyperparathyroidism. Endocrinology. 2008;149(11):5735–46.
9. Zingraff J, Drueke T, Marie P, Man NK, Jungers P, Bordier P. Anemia and secondary hyperparathyroidism. Arch Intern Med. 1978;138(11):1650–2.
10. Rao DS, Shih MS, Mohini R. Effect of serum parathyroid hormone and bone marrow fibrosis on the response to erythropoietin in uremia. N Engl J Med. 1993;328(3):171–5.
11. Meytes D, Bogin E, Ma A, Dukes PP, Massry SG. Effect of parathyroid hormone on erythropoiesis. J Clin Invest. 1981;67(5):1263–9.
12. Taniguchi S, Shibuya T, Harada M, Niho Y. Prostaglandin-mediated suppression of in vitro growth of erythroid progenitor cells. Kidney Int. 1989;36(4):712–8.
13. Dunn CD, Trent D. The effect of parathyroid hormone on erythropoiesis in serum-free cultures of fetal mouse liver cells. Proc Soc Exp Biol Med. 1981;166(4):556–61.
14. Komatsuda A, Hirokawa M, Haseyama T, Horiuchi T, Wakui H, Imai H, et al. Human parathyroid hormone does not influence human erythropoiesis in vitro. Nephrol Dial Transplant. 1998;13(8):2088–91.
15. Jacobson LO, Goldwasser E, Fried W, Plzak L. Role of the kidney in erythropoiesis. Nature. 1957;179(4560):633–4.
16. Naets JP. The role of the kidney in erythropoiesis. J Clin Invest. 1960;39:102–10.
17. Semenza GL, Wang GL. A nuclear factor induced by hypoxia via de novo protein synthesis binds to the human erythropoietin gene enhancer at a site required for transcriptional activation. Mol Cell Biol. 1992;12(12):5447–54.
18. Schodel J, Oikonomopoulos S, Ragoussis J, Pugh CW, Ratcliffe PJ, Mole DR. High-resolution genome-wide mapping of HIF-binding sites by ChIP-seq. Blood. 2011;117(23):e207–17.
19. Koury MJ, Haase VH. Anaemia in kidney disease: harnessing hypoxia responses for therapy. Nat Rev Nephrol. 2015;11(7):394–410.
20. Kobayashi H, Liu Q, Binns TC, Urrutia AA, Davidoff O, Kapitsinou PP, et al. Distinct subpopulations of FOXD1 stroma-derived cells regulate renal erythropoietin. J Clin Invest. 2016;126(5):1926–38.
21. Urena P, Eckardt KU, Sarfati E, Zingraff J, Zins B, Roullet JB, et al. Serum erythropoietin and erythropoiesis in primary and secondary hyperparathyroidism: effect of parathyroidectomy. Nephron. 1991;59(3):384–93.
22. Washio M, Iseki K, Onoyama K, Oh Y, Nakamoto M, Fujimi S, et al. Elevation of serum erythropoietin after subtotal parathyroidectomy in chronic haemodialysis patients. Nephrol Dial Transplant. 1992;7(2):121–4.
23. Borawski J, Pawlak K, Mysliwiec M. Inflammatory markers and platelet aggregation tests as predictors of hemoglobin and endogenous erythropoietin levels in hemodialysis patients. Nephron. 2002;91(4):671–81.
24. McGonigle RJ, Wallin JD, Husserl F, Deftos LJ, Rice JC, O'Neill WJ, et al. Potential role of parathyroid hormone as an inhibitor of erythropoiesis in the anemia of renal failure. J Lab Clin Med. 1984;104(6):1016–26.

25. Wong A, Loots GG, Yellowley CE, Dose AC, Genetos DC. Parathyroid hormone regulation of hypoxia-inducible factor signaling in osteoblastic cells. Bone. 2015;81:97–103.
26. Dunn MJ. Red blood cell calcium and magnesium: effects upon sodium and potassium transport and cellular morphology. Biochim Biophys Acta. 1974;352(1):97–116.
27. White JG. Effects of an ionophore, A23187, on the surface morphology of normal erythrocytes. Am J Pathol. 1974;77(3):507–18.
28. Weed RI, LaCelle PL, Merrill EW. Metabolic dependence of red cell deformability. J Clin Invest. 1969;48(5):795–809.
29. Lang E, Qadri SM, Lang F. Killing me softly - suicidal erythrocyte death. Int J Biochem Cell Biol. 2012;44(8):1236–43.
30. Bogin E, Massry SG, Levi J, Djaldeti M, Bristol G, Smith J. Effect of parathyroid hormone on osmotic fragility of human erythrocytes. J Clin Invest. 1982;69(4):1017–25.
31. Akmal M, Telfer N, Ansari AN, Massry SG. Erythrocyte survival in chronic renal failure. Role of secondary hyperparathyroidism. J Clin Invest. 1985;76(4):1695–8.
32. Barbour GL. Effect of parathyroidectomy on anemia in chronic renal failure. Arch Intern Med. 1979;139(8):889–91.
33. Mandolfo S, Malberti F, Farina M, Villa G, Scanziani R, Surian M, et al. Parathyroidectomy and response to erythropoietin therapy in anaemic patients with chronic renal failure. Nephrol Dial Transplant. 1998;13(10):2708–9.
34. Coen G, Calabria S, Bellinghieri G, Pecchini F, Conte F, Chiappini MG, et al. Parathyroidectomy in chronic renal failure: short- and long-term results on parathyroid function, blood pressure and anemia. Nephron. 2001;88(2):149–55.
35. Yasunaga C, Matsuo K, Yanagida T, Matsuo S, Nakamoto M, Goya T. Early effects of parathyroidectomy on erythropoietin production in secondary hyperparathyroidism. Am J Surg. 2002;183(2):199–204.
36. Trunzo JA, McHenry CR, Schulak JA, Wilhelm SM. Effect of parathyroidectomy on anemia and erythropoietin dosing in end-stage renal disease patients with hyperparathyroidism. Surgery. 2008;144(6):915–8; discussion 9.
37. Bhadada SK, Bhansali A, Ahluwalia J, Chanukya GV, Behera A, Dutta P. Anaemia and marrow fibrosis in patients with primary hyperparathyroidism before and after curative parathyroidectomy. Clin Endocrinol (Oxf). 2009;70(4):527–32.
38. Block GA, Bushinsky DA, Cunningham J, Drueke TB, Ketteler M, Kewalramani R, et al. Effect of Etelcalcetide vs. Placebo on Serum Parathyroid Hormone in Patients Receiving Hemodialysis With Secondary Hyperparathyroidism: Two Randomized Clinical Trials. JAMA. 2017;317(2):146–55.
39. Block GA, Bushinsky DA, Cheng S, Cunningham J, Dehmel B, Drueke TB, et al. Effect of etelcalcetide vs cinacalcet on serum parathyroid hormone in patients receiving hemodialysis with secondary hyperparathyroidism: a randomized clinical trial. JAMA. 2017;317(2):156–64.
40. Fukagawa M, Yokoyama K, Shigematsu T, Akiba T, Fujii A, Kuramoto T, et al. A phase 3, multicentre, randomized, double-blind, placebo-controlled, parallel-group study to evaluate the efficacy and safety of etelcalcetide (ONO-5163/AMG 416), a novel intravenous calcimimetic, for secondary hyperparathyroidism in Japanese haemodialysis patients. Nephrol Dial Transplant. 2017;32(10):1723–30.
41. Chertow GM, Block GA, Correa-Rotter R, Drueke TB, Floege J, Goodman WG, et al. Effect of cinacalcet on cardiovascular disease in patients undergoing dialysis. N Engl J Med. 2012;367(26):2482–94.
42. Moe SM, Chertow GM, Parfrey PS, Kubo Y, Block GA, Correa-Rotter R, et al. Cinacalcet, fibroblast growth Factor-23, and cardiovascular disease in hemodialysis: the evaluation of cinacalcet HCl therapy to lower cardiovascular events (EVOLVE) Ttrial. Circulation. 2015;132(1):27–39.
43. Battistella M, Richardson RM, Bargman JM, Chan CT. Improved parathyroid hormone control by cinacalcet is associated with reduction in darbepoetin requirement in patients with end-stage renal disease. Clin Nephrol. 2011;76(2):99–103.

44. Tanaka M, Yoshida K, Fukuma S, Ito K, Matsushita K, Fukagawa M, et al. Effects of secondary hyperparathyroidism treatment on improvement in anemia: results from the MBD-5D study. PLoS ONE. 2016;11(10):e0164865.

45. Albitar S, Genin R, Fen-Chong M, Serveaux MO, Schohn D, Chuet C. High-dose alfa-calcidol improves anaemia in patients on haemodialysis. Nephrol Dial Transplant. 1997;12(3):514–8.

46. Goicoechea M, Vazquez MI, Ruiz MA, Gomez-Campdera F, Perez-Garcia R, Valderrabano F. Intravenous calcitriol improves anaemia and reduces the need for erythropoietin in hae-modialysis patients. Nephron. 1998;78(1):23–7.

47. Singer RF. Vitamin D in dialysis: defining deficiency and rationale for supplementation. Semin Dial. 2013;26(1):40–6.

48. Kiss Z, Ambrus C, Almasi C, Berta K, Deak G, Horonyi P, et al. Serum 25(OH)-cholecalciferol concentration is associated with hemoglobin level and eryth-ropoietin resistance in patients on maintenance hemodialysis. Nephron Clin Pract. 2011;117(4):c373–8.

49. Rianthavorn P, Boonyapapong P. Ergocalciferol decreases erythropoietin resistance in chil-dren with chronic kidney disease stage 5. Pediatr Nephrol. 2013;28(8):1261–6.

50. Miskulin DC, Majchrzak K, Tighiouart H, Muther RS, Kapoian T, Johnson DS, et al. Ergocalciferol supplementation in hemodialysis patients with vitamin D deficiency: a rand-omized clinical trial. J Am Soc Nephrol. 2016;27(6):1801–10.

51. Marckmann P, Agerskov H, Thineshkumar S, Bladbjerg EM, Sidelmann JJ, Jespersen J, et al. Randomized controlled trial of cholecalciferol supplementation in chronic kidney dis-ease patients with hypovitaminosis D. Nephrol Dial Transplant. 2012;27(9):3523–31.

52. Verstuyf A, Carmeliet G, Bouillon R, Mathieu C. Vitamin D: a pleiotropic hormone. Kidney Int. 2010;78(2):140–5.

53. Cortes M, Chen MJ, Stachura DL, Liu SY, Kwan W, Wright F, et al. Developmental vitamin D availability impacts hematopoietic stem cell production. Cell Rep. 2016;17(2):458–68.

54. Calvi LM, Sims NA, Hunzelman JL, Knight MC, Giovannetti A, Saxton JM, et al. Activated parathyroid hormone/parathyroid hormone-related protein receptor in osteoblastic cells dif-ferentially affects cortical and trabecular bone. J Clin Invest. 2001;107(3):277–86.

55. Lord BI, Testa NG, Hendry JH. The relative spatial distributions of CFUs and CFUc in the normal mouse femur. Blood. 1975;46(1):65–72.

56. Taichman RS, Emerson SG. Human osteoblasts support hematopoiesis through the produc-tion of granulocyte colony-stimulating factor. J Exp Med. 1994;179(5):1677–82.

57. Calvi LM, Adams GB, Weibrecht KW, Weber JM, Olson DP, Knight MC, et al. Osteoblastic cells regulate the haematopoietic stem cell niche. Nature. 2003;425(6960):841–6.

58. Weber JM, Forsythe SR, Christianson CA, Frisch BJ, Gigliotti BJ, Jordan CT, et al. Parathyroid hormone stimulates expression of the Notch ligand Jagged1 in osteoblastic cells. Bone. 2006;39(3):485–93.

59. Chang SK, Noss EH, Chen M, Gu Z, Townsend K, Grenha R, et al. Cadherin-11 regulates fibroblast inflammation. Proc Natl Acad Sci USA. 2011;108(20):8402–7.

60. Yao H, Miura Y, Yoshioka S, Miura M, Hayashi Y, Tamura A, et al. Parathyroid hormone enhances hematopoietic expansion via upregulation of cadherin-11 in bone marrow mesen-chymal stromal cells. Stem Cells. 2014;32(8):2245–55.

61. Brunner S, Theiss HD, Murr A, Negele T, Franz WM. Primary hyperparathyroidism is associated with increased circulating bone marrow-derived progenitor cells. Am J Physiol Endocrinol Metab. 2007;293(6):E1670–5.

62. Yu EW, Kumbhani R, Siwila-Sackman E, DeLelys M, Preffer FI, Leder BZ, et al. Teriparatide (PTH 1-34) treatment increases peripheral hematopoietic stem cells in post-menopausal women. J Bone Miner Res. 2014;29(6):1380–6.

63. Ballen KK, Shpall EJ, Avigan D, Yeap BY, Fisher DC, McDermott K, et al. Phase I trial of parathyroid hormone to facilitate stem cell mobilization. Biol Blood Marrow Transplant. 2007;13(7):838–43.

64. Ballen KK, Cutler C, Yeap BY, McAfee SL, Dey BR, Attar EC, et al. Donor-derived second hematologic malignancies after cord blood transplantation. Biol Blood Marrow Transplant. 2010;16(7):1025–31.
65. Cahu X, Rialland F, Touzeau C, Chevallier P, Guillaume T, Delaunay J, et al. Infectious complications after unrelated umbilical cord blood transplantation in adult patients with hematologic malignancies. Biol Blood Marrow Transplant. 2009;15(12):1531–7.
66. de Lima M, McMannis J, Gee A, Komanduri K, Couriel D, Andersson BS, et al. Transplantation of ex vivo expanded cord blood cells using the copper chelator tetraethylenepentamine: a phase I/II clinical trial. Bone Marrow Transplant. 2008;41(9):771–8.
67. Delaney C, Heimfeld S, Brashem-Stein C, Voorhies H, Manger RL, Bernstein ID. Notch-mediated expansion of human cord blood progenitor cells capable of rapid myeloid reconstitution. Nat Med. 2010;16(2):232–6.
68. Ballen K, Mendizabal AM, Cutler C, Politikos I, Jamieson K, Shpall EJ, et al. Phase II trial of parathyroid hormone after double umbilical cord blood transplantation. Biol Blood Marrow Transplant. 2012;18(12):1851–8.
69. Fujita T, Inoue T, Morii H, Morita R, Norimatsu H, Orimo H, et al. Effect of an intermittent weekly dose of human parathyroid hormone (1-34) on osteoporosis: a randomized double-masked prospective study using three dose levels. Osteoporos Int. 1999;9(4):296–306.
70. Neer RM, Arnaud CD, Zanchetta JR, Prince R, Gaich GA, Reginster JY, et al. Effect of parathyroid hormone (1-34) on fractures and bone mineral density in postmenopausal women with osteoporosis. N Engl J Med. 2001;344(19):1434–41.
71. Sarnak MJ, Jaber BL. Mortality caused by sepsis in patients with end-stage renal disease compared with the general population. Kidney Int. 2000;58(4):1758–64.
72. Powe NR, Jaar B, Furth SL, Hermann J, Briggs W. Septicemia in dialysis patients: incidence, risk factors, and prognosis. Kidney Int. 1999;55(3):1081–90.
73. Plantinga LC, Fink NE, Melamed ML, Briggs WA, Powe NR, Jaar BG. Serum phosphate levels and risk of infection in incident dialysis patients. Clin J Am Soc Nephrol. 2008;3(5):1398–406.
74. Blayney MJ, Pisoni RL, Bragg-Gresham JL, Bommer J, Piera L, Saito A, et al. High alkaline phosphatase levels in hemodialysis patients are associated with higher risk of hospitalization and death. Kidney Int. 2008;74(5):655–63.
75. Young EW, Albert JM, Satayathum S, Goodkin DA, Pisoni RL, Akiba T, et al. Predictors and consequences of altered mineral metabolism: the Dialysis Outcomes and Practice Patterns Study. Kidney Int. 2005;67(3):1179–87.
76. Massry SG, Schaefer RM, Teschner M, Roeder M, Zull JF, Heidland A. Effect of parathyroid hormone on elastase release from human polymorphonuclear leucocytes. Kidney Int. 1989;36(5):883–90.
77. Doherty CC, LaBelle P, Collins JF, Brautbar N, Massry SG. Effect of parathyroid hormone on random migration of human polymorphonuclear leukocytes. Am J Nephrol. 1988;8(3):212–9.
78. Alexiewicz JM, Smogorzewski M, Fadda GZ, Massry SG. Impaired phagocytosis in dialysis patients: studies on mechanisms. Am J Nephrol. 1991;11(2):102–11.
79. Massry S, Smogorzewski M. Dysfunction of polymorphonuclear leukocytes in uremia: role of parathyroid hormone. Kidney Int Suppl. 2001;78:S195–6.
80. Horl WH, Haag-Weber M, Mai B, Massry SG. Verapamil reverses abnormal [Ca2+]i and carbohydrate metabolism of PMNL of dialysis patients. Kidney Int. 1995;47(6):1741–5.
81. Cho SW, Soki FN, Koh AJ, Eber MR, Entezami P, Park SI, et al. Osteal macrophages support physiologic skeletal remodeling and anabolic actions of parathyroid hormone in bone. Proc Natl Acad Sci USA. 2014;111(4):1545–50.
82. Gordon S, Pluddemann A, Martinez Estrada F. Macrophage heterogeneity in tissues: phenotypic diversity and functions. Immunol Rev. 2014;262(1):36–55.

83. Chang MK, Raggatt LJ, Alexander KA, Kuliwaba JS, Fazzalari NL, Schroder K, et al. Osteal tissue macrophages are intercalated throughout human and mouse bone lining tissues and regulate osteoblast function in vitro and in vivo. J Immunol. 2008;181(2):1232–44.

84. Perry HM 3rd, Chappel JC, Bellorin-Font E, Tamao J, Martin KJ, Teitelbaum SL. Parathyroid hormone receptors in circulating human mononuclear leukocytes. J Biol Chem. 1984;259(9):5531–5.

85. Alexiewicz JM, Klinger M, Pitts TO, Gaciong Z, Linker-Israeli M, Massry SG. Parathyroid hormone inhibits B cell proliferation: implications in chronic renal failure. J Am Soc Nephrol. 1990;1(3):236–44.

86. Gaciong Z, Alexiewicz JM, Linker-Israeli M, Shulman IA, Pitts TO, Massry SG. Inhibition of immunoglobulin production by parathyroid hormone. Implications in chronic renal failure. Kidney Int. 1991;40(1):96–106.

87. Gaciong Z, Alexiewicz JM, Massry SG. Impaired in vivo antibody production in CRF rats: role of secondary hyperparathyroidism. Kidney Int. 1991;40(5):862–7.

88. Kotzmann H, Koller M, Abela C, Clodi M, Riedl M, Graninger W, et al. Effects of parathyroid hormone and serum calcium on the phenotype and function of mononuclear cells in patients with primary hyperparathyroidism. Eur J Clin Invest. 1998;28(5):353–8.

89. Dominguez-Villar M, Hafler DA. Regulatory T cells in autoimmune disease. Nat Immunol. 2018;19(7):665–73.

90. Klinger M, Alexiewicz JM, Linker-Israeli M, Pitts TO, Gaciong Z, Fadda GZ, et al. Effect of parathyroid hormone on human T cell activation. Kidney Int. 1990;37(6):1543–51.

91. Tzanno-Martins C, Futata E, Jorgetti V, Duarte AJ. Restoration of impaired T-cell proliferation after parathyroidectomy in hemodialysis patients. Nephron. 2000;84(3):224–7.

92. Tokoyoda K, Egawa T, Sugiyama T, Choi BI, Nagasawa T. Cellular niches controlling B lymphocyte behavior within bone marrow during development. Immunity. 2004;20(6):707–18.

93. Zhu J, Garrett R, Jung Y, Zhang Y, Kim N, Wang J, et al. Osteoblasts support B-lymphocyte commitment and differentiation from hematopoietic stem cells. Blood. 2007;109(9):3706–12.

94. Wu JY, Purton LE, Rodda SJ, Chen M, Weinstein LS, McMahon AP, et al. Osteoblastic regulation of B lymphopoiesis is mediated by Gs{alpha}-dependent signaling pathways. Proc Natl Acad Sci U S A. 2008;105(44):16976–81.

95. Panaroni C, Fulzele K, Saini V, Chubb R, Pajevic PD, Wu JY. PTH signaling in osteoprogenitors is essential for B-lymphocyte differentiation and mobilization. J Bone Miner Res. 2015;30(12):2273–86.

96. Gao Y, Wu X, Terauchi M, Li JY, Grassi F, Galley S, et al. T cells potentiate PTH-induced cortical bone loss through CD40L signaling. Cell Metab. 2008;8(2):132–45.

97. Terauchi M, Li JY, Bedi B, Baek KH, Tawfeek H, Galley S, et al. T lymphocytes amplify the anabolic activity of parathyroid hormone through Wnt10b signaling. Cell Metab. 2009;10(3):229–40.

98. Bhadada SK, Sridhar S, Ahluwalia J, Bhansali A, Malhotra P, Behera A, et al. Anemia and thrombocytopenia improves after curative parathyroidectomy in a patient of primary hyperparathyroidism (PHPT). J Clin Endocrinol Metab. 2012;97(5):1420–2.

99. Ortega A, Perez de Prada MT, Mateos-Caceres PJ, Ramos Mozo P, Gonzalez-Armengol JJ, Gonzalez Del Castillo JM, et al. Effect of parathyroid-hormone-related protein on human platelet activation. Clin Sci (Lond). 2007;113(7):319–27.

100. Verdoia M, Pergolini P, Rolla R, Nardin M, Barbieri L, Schaffer A, et al. Parathyroid hormone levels and high-residual platelet reactivity in patients receiving dual antiplatelet therapy with acetylsalicylic acid and clopidogrel or ticagrelor. Cardiovasc Ther. 2016;34(4):209–15.

101. Watson PH, Fraher LJ, Hendy GN, Chung UI, Kisiel M, Natale BV, et al. Nuclear localization of the type 1 PTH/PTHrP receptor in rat tissues. J Bone Miner Res. 2000;15(6):1033–44.

102. Pringle A, Smith EK. Renal vein thrombosis in acute hyperthyroidism. Br Med J. 1964;2(5410):675–6.
103. Manosroi W, Wannasai K, Phimphilai M. Pulmonary embolism and subclavian vein thrombosis in a patient with parathyroid carcinoma: case report and review of literature. J Med Assoc Thai. 2015;98(9):925–33.
104. Erem C, Kocak M, Nuhoglu I, Yilmaz M, Ucuncu O. Increased plasminogen activator inhibitor-1, decreased tissue factor pathway inhibitor, and unchanged thrombin-activatable fibrinolysis inhibitor levels in patients with primary hyperparathyroidism. Eur J Endocrinol. 2009;160(5):863–8.
105. Farahnak P, Larfars G, Sten-Linder M, Nilsson IL. Mild primary hyperparathyroidism: vitamin D deficiency and cardiovascular risk markers. J Clin Endocrinol Metab. 2011;96(7):2112–8.
106. Elbers LPB, Wijnberge M, Meijers JCM, Poland DCW, Brandjes DPM, Fliers E, et al. Coagulation and fibrinolysis in hyperparathyroidism secondary to vitamin D deficiency. Endocr Connect. 2018;7(2):325–33.

Parathyroid Hormone as a Uremic Toxin

Victoria Vo and Stuart M. Sprague

In chronic kidney disease (CKD) uremia is an elevation of retained toxic metabolic by-products and other compounds in the body related to reduced renal function and ultimately can result in multi-organ dysfunction. This dysfunction is mediated by uremic toxins which can manifest in an array of physical symptoms or through pathophysiologic changes and dysfunction of various organ systems. There are many substances that become elevated in the blood as renal function declines, but not all of these may be associated with a level of organ dysfunction. When examining compounds found elevated in the blood of uremic patients for their potential as uremic toxins Koch's postulates in identifying causative agents of infectious disease can be applied in much the same manner as was done by Massry [1–3]. In this way, the Massry/Koch postulates for uremic toxins establishes a consistent applicable criteria to evaluate specific compounds for their uremic potential. These requirements for consideration as a uremic toxin include (1) chemically identifiable and quantifiable, (2) found in elevated levels in uremic serum compared to non-uremic serum, (3) elevated levels are associated with pathophysiologic symptoms or organ dysfunction, and (4) proven biological activity in ex vivo, in vivo, or in vitro studies which mimic concentrations found in uremic serum which reproduces the symptom or pathophysiologic organ dysfunction.

A database established in 1999 by researchers in Europe, the European Uremic Toxins (EUTox) Work Group, has propelled ongoing research for the "identification of yet unknown uremic toxins, the characterization of uremic toxins and the development of new therapeutic approaches for the treatment of chronic kidney

V. Vo
Division of Nephrology, Department of Medicine, University of Chicago Pritzker
School of Medicine, Chicago, IL, USA

S.M. Sprague (✉)
Division of Nephrology, Department of Medicine, North University Health System –
University of Chicago Pritzker School of Medicine, Evanston, IL, USA
e-mail: stuartmsprague@gmail.com

© Springer Nature Switzerland AG 2020
A. Covic et al. (eds.), *Parathyroid Glands in Chronic Kidney Disease*,
https://doi.org/10.1007/978-3-030-43769-5_9

diseases" [4]. This database utilizes criteria similar to the Massry/Koch postulate for the determination of a uremic toxin [5].

Uremic retention products are most often associated with low molecular weight toxic metabolites of protein and amino acids such as urea, guanidines, indoles, aromatic acids, aliphatic amines, aromatic amines, and peptides [1, 6]. In the clinical setting, blood urea nitrogen (BUN) is used as a surrogate marker for measuring these low molecular weight uremic retention products in the blood as well as determining both renal and dialytic clearance. Though urea is abundant in the blood and levels increase dramatically as renal function declines, it has a controversial history on whether it would classify as a uremic toxin. Prior human and animal model studies examining the effects of urea and its contribution to the uremic state have not shown that elevated levels of urea contribute to physical symptoms associated with uremia [7], but there remain concerns that urea likely plays an indefinable role in the uremic state [8].

Though many low molecular weight compounds have been theorized to significantly contribute into the uremic state, the middle molecular theory has identified many larger compounds (molecular weight > 500 Da and < 12,000 Da) which may also play a major role in uremic patients [2, 6]. Among these middle molecules is parathyroid hormone (PTH), which is elevated in CKD patients due to excess endogenous production, decreased degradation and impaired renal clearance of the hormone [9].

Put forth by Massry [1], PTH meets all the criteria outline by Koch and the EUTox Work Groupas a uremic toxin. Not only does PTH contribute to bone and mineral dysfunction in CKD patients but this hormone acts as a uremic toxin to many other organ systems (Table 1). It can affect many systems in the body in ways that are unexpected, varying widely from known effects of PTH predominantly centered on bone and mineral homeostasis. Though the effects of PTH on these different organ systems is surprising, most effects are still predominately mediated through calcium regulation within these systems.

Although PTH affects numerous organ systems as a uremic toxin, its role in anemia, soft tissue necrosis, and cardiovascular disease are of the most prominent uremic complications in CKD patients. It is important to understand how PTH influences these processes as each are complicated disease processes which are influenced by many pathological pathways to which PTH contributes.

Anemia in CKD patients is predominantly associated with impaired erythropoietin production and response. Studies have found that elevated serum PTH has a direct inhibitory effect on erythroid colony growth [21], indirectly effects erythropoiesis via bone marrow fibrosis seen in secondary hyperparathyroidism [22], and also directly effects red blood cells (RBC) by increasing osmotic fragility resulting in reduced life span of uremic RBCs [20]. Additionally, PTH affects other hematologic components including leukocytes. Animal model studies have shown that PTH acts upon polymorphonuclear leukocytes and reduces phagocytosis [19], and in vitro models have found PTH decreases T lymphocyte proliferation and production of B lymphocytes [18].

Table 1 Pathophysiologic manifestations of uremia mediated by elevated PTH

	Pathophysiologic effects on organ systems by elevated PTH
Musculoskeletal	Muscular weakness—decreased mitochondrial activity in skeletal muscle and reduced amino acid and fatty acid metabolism [10–12] Renal osteodystrophy—direct activation of osteoblasts, stimulation of OPG-RANKL signaling pathway, cellular apoptosis [13]
Cardiovascular	Cardiac fibrosis—increased intracellular calcium of cardiomyocytes leading to increased beat rate and early cell death [14] and cardiac fibroblast activation [15] Vascular calcification—high calcium phosphate product [16]
Pulmonary	Pulmonary hypertension—pulmonary calcification [17]
Hematologic	Depressed immunologic response—decrease cellular proliferation of T lymphocytes, reduced production of B lymphocytes [18], and impaired phagocytosis [19] Anemia—increased intracellular calcium in red blood cells can affect their integrity and induce hemolysis [20]; modulation of erythropoiesis through bone marrow fibrosis [21, 22]
Nervous	Encephalopathy—increased calcium concentration in gray and white matter of the brain [23, 24] Peripheral neuropathy—decreased motor nerve conduction velocity mediated through increased nerve calcium levels [25, 26]
Endocrine	Glucose intolerance—PTH mediated decrease in insulin secretion by beta cells [27, 28] Hyperlipidemia/hypertriglyceridemia—downregulation of hepatic tissue lipoprotein lipase [29, 30]
Integumentary	Pruritus—likely via high calcium phosphorus product [31–34]
Soft Tissue	Calcific uremic arteriopathy/calciphylaxis [35–37]

A major complication of uremia is soft tissue necrosis which is a result of high calcium phosphate products and vascular calcification associated with tissue ischemia, also known as calciphylaxis or calcific uremic arteriolopathy [37]. Case studies have shown that despite low calcium phosphate products these lesions could still persists after renal transplant in the setting of tertiary hyperparathyroidism and elevated PTH. This suggests an independent role for PTH in the development and maintenance of these lesions [35–37], and a possible answer as to why some develop calciphylaxis and others do not. Beyond soft tissue necrosis, high calcium phosphate products also contribute to pulmonary calcifications which may contribute to pulmonary hypertension [17] and pruritus. Pruritus is a uremic symptom that plagues advanced CKD and end stage renal disease (ESRD) patients. Though the exact mechanism is not clear, high calcium phosphate product is speculated to contribute to the development of pruritus as this symptom has been seen to improve and sometimes resolve after parathyroidectomy [31–34].

An important pathophysiologic effect of PTH as a uremic toxin is it role in cardiac fibrosis. Animal studies have found that elevated PTH concentrations cause selective activation of cardiac fibroblasts which then generate intermyocardiocyte fibrosis with collage deposition [15]. In addition, other animal have shown that elevated PTH levels stimulated and increased rate of beating in cardiac cells as well as causing earlier cellular death of these cells [14]. This is important insight into how elevated PTH contributes to increased morbidity and mortality in ESRD patients.

Beyond the direct uremic effects caused by PTH on various organ systems, hyperparathyroidism is central to the mineral dysfunction associated with chronic kidney disease-bone and mineral disorder (CKD-MBD) and has been shown to contribute significantly to morbidity and cardiovascular mortality in CKD and ESRD patients [38]. As renal function declines in CKD there is total body retention of phosphate and ultimately decrease in serum calcium concentrations. The physiologic/hormonal mechanisms to maintain normal mineral homeostasis ultimately fails. The changes in mineral metabolism with the development of CKD involves marked increases of PTH and fibroblast growth factor 23 (FGF23), with significant decreases in klotho and calcitriol [39]. These mechanisms have been described as the PTH-Vitamin D-FGF23 axis [40] or the FGF23-PTH endocrine loop [41].

FGF23 is produced principally by osteocytes and osteoblasts to act as an endocrine hormone capable of regulating serum phosphate, calcium, 1,25-dihydroxyvitamin D, and PTH. FGF23 acting on its receptor complex, klotho-FGFR1, located in the parathyroid gland results in down regulation of PTH gene expression, decreased PTH secretion, and decreased parathyroid cell proliferation [42]. In both human and animal models, iatrogenic elevation of PTH levels have resulted in the development of increased serum FGF23 concentrations, and after parathyroidectomy in animal models the elevation of FGF23 is corrected [43, 44]. The results of these studies indicate that PTH plays a stimulatory role FGF23 secretion. The apparent PTH stimulation of FGF23 secretion and FGF23 negative feedback on PTH secretion completes a bone parathyroid hormonal axis [41].

There also has been studies that show a positive correlation between 1,25-dihydroxyvitamin D levels and FGF23 levels where increasing serum levels of 1,25-dihydroxyvitamin D simulates elevated levels of FGF23 [45, 46]. FGF23 in turn acts upon its klotho-FGFR1 receptor complex in the kidney which has been found to decrease production of 1,25-dihydroxyvitamin D by suppressing the action of 1 α-hydroxylase and stimulation of 24-hydroxylase [47, 48]. This is opposite of the effect PTH has on the kidney as it increases 1,25-dihydroxyvitamin D production, which then in turn suppresses PTH production by the parathyroid gland. This cycle of positive and negative feedback comprises the PTH-Vitamin D-FGF23 axis.

FGF23 is also involved in the regulation of serum phosphate. Several studies evaluating elevated serum phosphate, via loading of both enteral and parenteral phosphate, have revealed increases in FGF23 associated with the rise in serum phosphate [49, 50] and that serum phosphate levels also acts as a key regulator for FGF23 secretion by bone. FGF23, acting on its klotho-FGFR1 receptor complex in the kidney, reduces phosphate reabsorption by the kidney through down regulation of NaPi-2a cotransporters on the apical side of the proximal tubule [47] thereby causing hyperphosphaturia and decreases serum phosphate.

Outside of the effect on bone mineral disease in CKD patients, serum FGF23 has also been found to be a uremic toxin. As renal function declines serum FGF23 rises in response to the increasingly elevated serum phosphate and PTH concentrations. Elevated serum FGF23 has been associated with cardiomyocyte hypertrophy [51] and left ventricular hypertrophy, which ultimately promotes diastolic dysfunction, congestive heart failure, and arrhythmias [52, 53]. The mechanism by which FGF23 acts upon the heart is through FGFR4, a receptor that is not coupled with klotho as found in other FGF23 target organs [51]. Through its actions on the heart and the disturbances on cardiac function, FGF23 increases cardiovascular mortality in the CKD and ESRD population [52, 54].

In summary, PTH is a uremic toxin with multiple systemic effects including myopathy, neurologic abnormalities, anemia, pruritus, cardiomyopathy, and the is the primary cause of the mineral metabolism dysfunction associated with CKD-MBD. These disorders results in significant morbidity and mortality if left untreated. Thus, clinical practice guidelines recommend frequent measurement in order to determine trends and implement appropriate treatments.

References

1. Massry SG. Is parathyroid hormone a uremic toxin? Nephron. 1977;17:125–30.
2. Glassock R. Uremic toxins: What are they? An integrated overview of pathobiology and classification. J Renal Nutr. 2008;18(1):2–6.
3. Dobre M, Meyer TW, Hostetter TH. Searching for uremic toxins. Clin J Am Soc Nephrol. 2013;8(2):322–7.
4. Retrieved November 28, 2010, from http://www.uremic-toxins.org.
5. Vanholder R, Argiles A, Baurmeister U, Brunet P, Clark W, Cohen G, DeDeyn PP, Deppisch R, Descamps-Latscha B, Henle T, Jorres A, Massy ZA, Rodroguez M, Stegmayr B, Stenvinkel P, Wratten ML. Uremic toxicity: present state of the art. Int J Artif Organs. 2001;24:695–725.
6. Barreto FC, Stinghen AEM, Oliveria RB, Franco ATB, Moreno AN, Barreto DV, Peoits-Filho R, Drueke TB, Massy ZA. The quest for a better understanding of chronic kidney disease complications: an update on uremic toxins. J Bras Nefrol. 2014;36(2):221–35.
7. Depner TA. Uremic toxicity: urea and beyond. Semin Dial. 2001;14(4):246–51.
8. Lau WL, Vaziri ND. Urea, a true uremic toxin: the empire strikes back. Clin Sci. 2016;131:3–12.
9. Slatopolsky E, Martin K, Hruska K. Parathyroid hormone metabolism and its potential as a uremic toxin. Am J Physiol. 1980;239(8):F1–12.
10. Baczynski R, Massry SG, Magott M, et al. Effect of parathyroid hormone on energy metabolism of skeletal muscle. Kidney Int. 1985;28:722–7.
11. Garber AJ. Effect of parathyroid hormone on skeletal muscle protein and amino acid metabolism in the rat. J Clin Invest. 1983;71:1806–L821.
12. Smogorzewski M, Pisorska G, Borum P, et al.: Chronic renal failure, parathyroid hormone and fatty acids oxidations in skeletal muscle. Kidney Int. 1988;33:555–60.
13. Sprague SM, Moe SM. The case for routine parathyroid hormone monitoring. Clin J Am Soc Nephrol. 2013;8:313–8.
14. Bogin E, Massry SG, Harary I. Effect of parathyroid hormone on rat heart cells. J Clin Invest. 1981;67(4):1215–27.
15. Amann K, Ritz E, Wiest G, Klaus G, Mall G. A role of parathyroid hormone for the activation of cardiac fibroblasts in uremia. J Am Soc Nephrol. 1994;4(10):1814–9.

16. ContigugliaSR, Alfrey AC, Miller NL, et al.: Nature of soft tissue calcification in uremia. Kidney Int 4:229-235, 1973.
17. Akmal M, Barmdt RR, Ansari AN, Mohler JG, Massry SG. Excess PTH in CRF induces pulmonary calcifications, pulmonary hypertension and right ventricular hypertrophy. Kidney Int. 1995;47(1):158–67.
18. Klinger M, Alexiewicz JM, Linker-Israeli M, Pitts TO, Gaciong Z, Fadda GZ, Massry SG. Effect of parathyroid hormone on human T cell activation. Kidney Int. 1990;37(6):1543–51.
19. Chervu I, Kiersztejn M, Alexiewicz JM, Fadda GZ, Smogorzewski M, Massry SG. Impaired phagocytosis in chronic renal failure is medicated by secondary hyperparathyroidism. Kidney Int. 1992;41(6):1501–5.
20. Bogin E, Massry SG, Levi J, Djaldeti M, Bristol G, Smith J. Effect of parathyroid hormone on osmotic fragility of human erythrocytes. J Clin Invest. 1982;69(4):1017–25.
21. Meytes D, Bogin E, Ma A, Dukes PP, Massry SG. Effect of parathyroid hormone on erythropoiesis. J Clin Invest. 1981;67(5):1263–9.
22. Rao DS, Shih MS, Mohini R. Effect of serum parathyroid hormone and bone marrow fibrosis on the response to erythropoietin in uremia. N Engl J Med. 1993;328(3):171–5.
23. Fuisado R, Arieff AI, Massry SG, Lazarowitz V, Kerian A. Changes in the electroencephalogram in acute uremia. Effects of parathyroid hormone and brain electrolytes. J Clin Invest. 1975;55:738–45.
24. Akmal M, Goldstein DA, Multani S, Massry SG. Role of uremia, brain calcium, and parathyroid hormone on changes in electroencephalogram in chronic renal failure. Am J Physiol. 1984;246:F575–9.
25. Avram MM, Feinfeld DA, Huatuco AH. Search for the uremic toxin decreased motor-nerve conduction velocity and elevated parathyroid hormone in uremia. NEJM. 1978;298(18):1000–3.
26. Goldstein DA, Chui LA, Massry SG. Effect of parathyroid hormone and uremia on peripheral nerve calcium and motor nerve conduction velocity. J Clin Investi. 1978;62(1):88–93.
27. Akmal M, Massry SG, Goldstein DA, Fanti P, Weisz A, DeFronzo RA. Role of parathyroid hormone in the glucose intolerance of chronic renal failure. J Clin Invest. 1985;75(3):1037–44.
28. Mak RH, Betttinelli A, Turner C, Haycock GB, Chantler C. The influence of hyperparathyroidism on glucose metabolism in uremia. J Clin Endocrinol Metab. 1985;60:229–33.
29. Lacour B, Roullet JB, Liagre AM, Jorgetti V, Beyne P, Dubost C, Drueke T. Serum lipoprotein disturbances in primary and secondary hyperparathyroidism and effects of parathyroidectomy. Am J Kidney Dis. 1986;8(6):422–9.
30. Klin M, Smogorzewki M, Ni Z, Zhang G, Massry SG. Abnormalities in hepatic lipase in chronic renal failure role of excess parathyroid hormone. J Clin Invest. 1996;97(10):2167–73.
31. Massry SG, Popovtzer MM, Coburn JW, et al. Intractable pruritus as a manifestation of secondary hyperparathyroidism in uremia. N EnglJMed. 1968;279:697–700.
32. Chou FF, Ho JC, Huang SC, Sheen-Chen SM. A study on pruritus after parathyroidectomy for secondary hyperparathyroidism. J Am Coll Surg. 2000;190(1):65–70.
33. Tajbakhsh R, Joshaghani HR, Bayzayi F, Haddad M, Qorbani M. Association between pruritus and serum concentrations of parathormone, calcium and phosphorus in hemodialysis patients. Saudi J Kidney Dis Transpl. 2013;24(4):702–6.
34. Makhlough A, Emadi N, Sedighi O, Khademloo M, Bicmohamadi AR. Relationship between serum intact parathyroid hormone and pruritus in hemodialysis patients. Iran J Kidney Dis. 2013;7(1):42–6.
35. Massry SG, Gordon A, Coburn JW, Kaplan L, Franklin SS, Maxwell MH, Kleeman CR. Vascular calcification and peripheral necrosis in a renal transplant recipient. Am J Med. 1970;49(3):416–22.
36. Richardson JA, Herron G, Reitz R, Layzer R. Ischemic ulcerations of skin and necrosis of muscle in azotemic hyperparathyroidism. Ann Intern Med. 1969;71(1):129–38.
37. Sprague SM. Painful skin ulcers in a hemodialysis patient. Clin J Am Soc Neph. 2014;9:166–173. [Epub ahead of print] PMID:24202137.

38. El Hilali J, de Koning EJ, van Ballegooijen AJ, Lips P, Sohl E, van Marwijk HWJ, Visser M, van Schoor NM. Vitamin D, PTH and the risk of overall and disease specific mortality: Results of the longitudinal aging study Amsterdam. J Steroid Biochem Mol Biol. 2016;164:386–94.

39. Pavik I, Jaeger P, Ebner L, Wagner CA, Petzold K, Spichtig D, Poster D, Wuthrich P, Russman S, Serra AL. Secreted klotho and FGF23 in chronic kidney disease stage 1 to 5: a sequence suggested from a cross-sectional study. Nepho Dial Transpl. 2013;28:352–9. https://doi.org/10.1093/ndt/gfs460.

40. Blau JE, Colllins MT. The PTH-Vitamin D-FGF23 axis. Rev Endocr Metab Disord. 2015;16:165–74.

41. Silver J, Rodriguez M, Slatopolsky E. FGF23 and PTH-double agents at the heart of CKD. Nephrol Dial Transplant. 2012;27:1715–20.

42. Ben Dov IZ, Galitzer H, Lavi-Moshayoff V, Goetz R, Kuro-o M, Muhammadi M, Sirkis R, Naveh-Many T, Silver J. The parathyroid is a target organ for FGF23 in rats. J Clin Invest. 2007;117(12):4003–8.

43. Lavi-Moshayoff V, Wasserman G, Meir T, Silver J, Naveh-Many T. PTH increases FGF23 gene expression and mediates the high-FGF23 levels of experimental kidney failure: a bone parathyroid feedback loop. Am J Physio Renal Physio. 2010;299(4):F882–9.

44. Burnett-Bowie SA, Henao MP, Dere ME, Lee H, Leder BZ. Effects of hPTH(1-34) infusion on circulating serum phosphate, 1,25-dihydroxyvitamin D, and FGF23 levels in healthy men. J Bone Miner Res. 2009;24(10):1681–5.

45. Collins MT, Lindsay JR, Jain A, Kelly MH, Cutler CM, Weinstein LS, Liu J, Fedarko NS, Winer KK. Fibroblast growth factor-23 is regulated by 1alpha, 25 dihydroxyvitamin D. J Bone Miner Res. 2005;20(11):1944–50.

46. Nishi H, Nii-Kono T, Nakanishi S, Yamazaki Y, Yamashita T, Fukumoto S, Ikeda K, Fujimon A, Fukagawa M. Intravenous calcitriol therapy increases serum concentrations of fibroblast growth factor 23 in dialysis patients with secondary hyperparathyroidism. Nephron Clin Pract. 2005;101(2):c94–9.

47. Saito H, Kusano K, Kinosaki M, Ito H, Hirata M, Segawa H, Miyamoto K, Fukushima N. Human fibroblast growth factor-23 mutants suppress Na+-dependent phosphate co-transport activity and 1alpha, 25-dihydroxyvitamin D3 production. J Biol Chem. 2003;278(4):2206–11.

48. Shimada T, Kakitani M, Yamazaki Y, Hasegawa H, Takeuchi Y, Fujita T, Fukumoto S, Tomizuka K, Yamashita T. Targeted ablation of FGF23 demonstrates an essential physiological role of FGF23 in phosphate and vitamin D metabolism. J Clin Invest. 2004;113(4):561–8.

49. Burnett SM, Gunawardene SC, Bringhurst FR, Juppner H, Lee H, Finkelstein JS. Regulation of C-terminal and intact FGF-23 by dietary phosphate in men and women. J Bone Miner Res. 2006;21(8):1187–96.

50. Scanni R, vonRotz M, Jehle S, Hulter HN, Krapf R. The human response to acute enteral and parenteral phosphate loads. J Am Soc Nephrol. 2014;25(12):2730–9.

51. Leifheit-Nestler M, Grabner A, Hermann L, Ritcher B, Schmitz K, Fischer DC, Yanucil C, Faul C, Haffner D. Vitamin D treatment attenuates cardiac FGF23/FGFR4 signaling and hypertrophy in uremic rats. Nephrol Dial Transplant. 2017;32:1493–503.

52. Isakova T, Xie H, Yang W, Xie D, Anderson AH, Scialla J, Wahl P, Gutiérrez OM, Steigerwalt S, He J, Schwartz S, Lo J, Ojo A, Sondheimer J, Hsu CY, Lash J, Leonard M, Kusek JW, Feldman HI, Wolf M. Fibroblast growth factor 23 and risks of mortality and end-stage renal disease in patients with chronic kidney disease. JAMA. 2011;305(23):2432–3439.

53. Glassock RJ, Pecoits-Filho R, Barberato SH. Left ventricular mass in chronic kidney disease and ESRD. Clin J Am Soc Nephrol. 2009;4:S79–91.

54. Wolf M. Update on fibroblast growth factor 23 in chronic kidney disease. Kidney Int. 2012;82(7):737–47.

Control of Secondary Hyperparathyroidism (SPHT) by Older and Newer Vitamin D Compounds

David Goldsmith

True deficiency, or relative insufficiency, of 25-hydroxyvitamin D (25-OHD)—and consequentially, deficiency of 1,25 di-OH vitamin D—are highly prevalent among patients with chronic kidney disease (CKD) or end-stage renal disease (ESRD) and these are critical components, together with chronic hyperphosphataemia, in the pathogenesis of SHPT. Accordingly, current guidelines have chosen to recommend the correction of hypovitaminosis D through nutritional vitamin D replacement [1, 2], though this is decidedly NOT evidenced based, more an expression of optimism that the many "pleiotropic" claimed effects of vitamin D repletion—reduction in cardiovascular disease, infection and cancer—would somehow apply to renal patients as well. A crunching, crushing hammer blow to the concept of "the sunshine vitamin" somehow protecting general health if only repleted/replaced has been dealt by the final publication of the very-long awaited study, VITAL: in this huge US-based study, a total of 25,871 participants, including 5106 black participants, underwent randomisation. Supplementation with vitamin D was not associated with a lower risk of either of the cardiovascular or cancer primary end points. During a median follow-up of 5.3 years, cancer was diagnosed in 1617 participants (793 in the vitamin D group and 824 in the placebo group; hazard ratio, 0.96; 95% confidence interval [CI], 0.88–1.06; $P=0.47$). A major cardiovascular event occurred in 805 participants (396 in the vitamin D group and 409 in the placebo group; hazard ratio, 0.97; 95% CI, 0.85–1.12; $P=0.69$). In the analyses of secondary end points, the hazard ratios were as follows: for death from cancer (341 deaths), 0.83 (95% CI, 0.67–1.02); for breast cancer, 1.02 (95% CI, 0.79–1.31); for prostate cancer, 0.88 (95% CI, 0.72–1.07); for colorectal cancer, 1.09 (95% CI, 0.73–1.62); for the expanded composite end point of major cardiovascular events plus coronary revascularization, 0.96 (95% CI, 0.86–1.08); for myocardial infarction, 0.96 (95% CI, 0.78–1.19); for stroke, 0.95 (95% CI, 0.76–1.20); and for death from cardiovascular causes, 1.11 (95% CI, 0.88–1.40). In the

D. Goldsmith (✉)
Renal Unit at Guy's and St. Thomas' NHS Foundation Hospital, London, UK
e-mail: djagoldsmith@gmail.com

© Springer Nature Switzerland AG 2020
A. Covic et al. (eds.), *Parathyroid Glands in Chronic Kidney Disease*,
https://doi.org/10.1007/978-3-030-43769-5_10

analysis of death from any cause (978 deaths), the hazard ratio was 0.99 (95% CI, 0.87–1.12). No excess risks of hypercalcaemia or other adverse events were identified [3].

As deficiency of 25-hydroxyvitamin D (25[OH]D) is common in patients with CKD stages 3 and 4 and is consistently associated with poor outcomes, it may seem surprising that a "controversies conference" on vitamin D in chronic kidney disease was sponsored by the National Kidney Foundation in 2017, reporting in 2018 [4]. The reason for this is that there is controversy and a lack of standardisation with respect to definition of vitamin D concentrations to be considered, optimal, adequate, insufficient or deficient in CKD. The report outlines the deliberations of the 3 work groups that participated in the conference. Until newer measurement methods are widely used, the panel agreed that clinicians should classify 25(OH)D "adequacy" as concentrations >20 ng/mL without evidence of counter-regulatory hormone activity (i.e., elevated PTH). The panel also agreed that 25(OH)D concentrations <15 ng/mL should be treated irrespective of PTH concentrations. Patients with 25(OH)D concentrations between 15 and 20 ng/mL may not require treatment if there is no evidence of counter-regulatory hormone activity (no elevation in PTH). The panel agreed that nutritional vitamin D (cholecalciferol, ergocalciferol, or calcifediol) should be supplemented before giving activated vitamin D compounds. The compounds need further study evaluating important outcomes that observational studies have linked to low 25(OH)D levels, such as progression to end-stage kidney disease, infections, fracture rates, hospitalizations, and all-cause mortality [5].

Sadly, implicit in these learned deliberations is a touching naivety that the sporadic measurement of serum/plasma PTH is reliable way to inform clinicians about skeletal health and integrity. This has been repeatedly shown not to be the case; algorithms must adapt to include the use of other biomarkers, including bone specific alkaline phosphatase [6–9].

Whereas nutritional vitamin D replacement may well easily restore 25-OHD concentration to near, or even above the "normal" range in health, the real target of treating vitamin D insufficiency **is and will always remain** the successful treatment of SHPT, which is thought to be immune to modulation (if solely defined by PTH concentrations, a poor substitute of course for proper holistic clinical care) by nutritional vitamin D [10]. Thus, while it is also the subject of a tacit recommendation by guidelines groups, it has also been stridently asserted that, there is little, if any, clinical utility or benefit of nutritional vitamin D replacement in CKD.

Ranged against that is softer evidence for the usefulness of using vitamin D to treat 'renal bone disease' which has been clinical custom and practice now for nearly six decades. In regular clinical practice, however, it is more like three decades, at most, that we have routinely been using vitamin D to try to prevent, or reverse, the impact of SHPT on the skeleton of patients with CKD. The practice has been in the main to use high doses of synthetic vitamin D compounds, not naturally occurring ones. However, the pharmacological impacts of the different vitamin D species and of their different modes, and styles of administration cannot be assumed to be uniform across the spectrum. It is disappointingly true to say that even in 2020 there is a remarkable, unacceptable and distressing paucity of evidence concerning the clinical benefits of vitamin D supplementation to treat vitamin D insufficiency in patients with stage 3b–5 CKD.

While there are a number of studies that report the impact of vitamin D supplementation on serum vitamin D concentrations (unsurprisingly, usually reporting a robust increase), and some variable evidence of serum PTH concentration suppression, there has been much less focus on hard or semi-rigid clinical end point analysis (e.g. fractures, hospitalizations and overall mortality). Now, in 2020, with the practice pattern changes of first widespread clinical use of vitamin D and second widespread supplementation of cholecalciferol or ergocalciferol by patients (alone, or as multivitamins), it is now, in my view, next to impossible to run a placebo-controlled trial over a decent period of time, especially one which involved clinically meaningful end-points, such as fractures, hospitalization, parathyroidectomy, and death. In this challenging situation, we need to ask what it is we are trying to achieve here, and how best to balance potential benefits with potential harm.

A recent and interesting development has occurred which has served to blur the false dichotomy between opponents and proponents of the use of nutritional vitamin D in CKD. Extended-release calcifediol (ERC) 30 μg capsules were recently approved by the United States Food and Drug Administration (FDA) for the treatment of SHPT in adults with stage 3–4 (not 5) CKD and vitamin D insufficiency (serum total 25OHD <75 nmol/L) [12]. Calcifediol is 25-hydroxyvitamin D3, a prohormone of the active calcitriol (1,25-dihydroxyvitamin D3). ERC capsules have a lipophilic fill, which gradually releases calcifediol, corrects vitamin D insufficiency, and increases serum calcitriol and thereby suppresses production of PTH in CKD patients without seeming to perturb normal vitamin D and mineral metabolism. Randomized clinical trials (RCTs) have demonstrated that non-modified nutritional vitamin D is ineffective for treating SHPT (when used in conventional doses, up to the equivalent of around 4000 IU/day) whereas vitamin D receptor activators (VDRA) can very easily and significantly correct elevated PTH concentrations, but with a marked increased risk of hypercalcaemia and hyperphosphataemia [11, 12], which has led KDIGO to suggest these VDRA drugs should not be used in CKD stages 3,4,5ND.

ERC might seem to offer healthcare professionals a new treatment option that has been demonstrated in RCTs to be safe and effective for controlling SHPT without clinically meaningfully increasing serum concentrations of calcium or phosphorus (at least in tested dosing, in clinical trial subjects, with up to 12 months follow-up). This development might therefore quite literally bridge the two positions. The stricture of the need to demonstrate with hard end-points (fractures, survival, patient-reported outcome measures) that there is any demonstrable benefit from so doing remains as compelling and urgent as ever [11, 12].

References

1. KDIGO. KDIGO clinical practice guideline for the diagnosis, evaluation, prevention, and treatment of Chronic Kidney Disease-Mineral and Bone Disorder (CKD-MBD). Kidney Int Suppl 2009(113):S1–130.
2. National Kidney F. K/DOQI clinical practice guidelines for bone metabolism and disease in chronic kidney disease. Am J Kidney Dis. 2003;42(4 Suppl 3):S1–201.
3. Manson JE, Cook NR, Lee IM, Christen W, Bassuk SS, Mora S, Gibson H, Gordon D,Copeland T, D'Agostino D, Friedenberg G, Ridge C, Bubes V, Giovannucci EL, Willett WC, Buring JE; VITAL Research Group. Vitamin D supplements and prevention of cancer and cardiovascular disease. N Engl J Med. 20193;380(1):33–44.
4. Melamed ML, Chonchol M, Gutiérrez OM, Kalantar-Zadeh K, Kendrick J, Norris K, Scialla JJ, Thadhani R. The role of vitamin D in CKD Stages 3 to 4: Report of a scientific workshop sponsored by the National Kidney Foundation. Am J Kidney Dis. 2018;72(6):834–845.).
5. O'Flaherty D, Sankaralingam A, Scully P, Manghat P, Goldsmith D, Hampson G. The relationship between intact PTH and biointact PTH (1-84) with bone and mineral metabolism in pre-dialysis chronic kidney disease (CKD). Clin Biochem. 2013;46(15):1405–9.
6. Sardiwal S, Magnusson P, Goldsmith DJ, Lamb EJ. Bone alkaline phosphatase in CKD-mineral bone disorder. Am J Kidney Dis. 2013;62(4):810–22.
7. Fernández-Martín JL, Carrero JJ, Benedik M, Bos WJ, Covic A, Ferreira A, Floege J, Goldsmith D, Gorriz JL, Ketteler M, Kramar R, Locatelli F, London G, Martin PY, Memmos D, Nagy J, Naves-Díaz M, Pavlovic D, Rodríguez-García M, Rutkowski B, Teplan V, Tielemans C, Verbeelen D, Wüthrich RP, Martínez-Camblor P, Cabezas-Rodriguez I, Sánchez-Alvarez JE, Cannata-Andia JB. COSMOS: the dialysis scenario of CKD-MBD in Europe. Nephrol Dial Transplant. 2013;28(7):1922–35.
8. Garrett G, Sardiwal S, Lamb EJ, Goldsmith DJ. PTH–a particularly tricky hormone: why measure it at all in kidney patients? Clin J Am Soc Nephrol. 2013;8(2):299–312.
9. Agarwal R, Georgianos PI. Con: Nutritional vitamin D replacement in chronic kidney disease and end-stage renal disease. Nephrol Dial Transplant. 2016;31(5):706–13.
10. Goldsmith DJ. Pro: Should we correct vitamin D deficiency/insufficiency in chronic kidney disease patients with inactive forms of vitamin D or just treat them with active vitamin D forms? Nephrol Dial Transplant. 2016;31(5):698–705.
11. Sprague SM, Crawford PW, Melnick JZ, et al. Use of extended-release calcifediol to treat secondary hyperparathyroidism in Stages 3 and 4 chronic kidney disease. Am J Nephrol. 2016;44(4):316–25.
12. Sprague SM, Strugnell SA, W. Bishop CW. Extended-release calcifediol (Rayaldee) for secondary hyperparathyroidism. Med Lett Drugs Ther. 2017;59(1515):36–37.

The Role of the Old and the New Calcimimetic Agents in Chronic Kidney Disease-Mineral and Bone Disorder

Luciano Pereira and João M. Frazão

Introduction

Chronic kidney disease (CKD) is an increasingly disease and a public health issue, affecting 8–16% of the population worldwide [1]. During the course of CKD, the decline of renal function leads to the development of calcium and phosphate metabolism disorders, causing a condition—"Mineral Bone Disease associated with CKD" (CKD-MBD) [2]. This condition develops with the incapacity of the kidney to excrete phosphate properly, leading to its retention and accumulation. Phosphate load stimulates Fibroblast Growth Factor 23 (FGF-23) and serum parathyroid hormone (PTH) [3]. FGF-23, a peptide hormone produced mainly in the osteocytes, is able to reduce phosphate levels using three different pathways: decreasing tubular epithelial cells reabsorption with the subsequent increase in renal excretion, stimulating PTH secretion with its additional phosphaturic effect

---

In preparation of this book chapter, we used previously published material, with permission (Licence number 4463751218679)—Review Paper "Old and new calcimimetics for treatment of secondary hyperparathyroidism: impact on biochemical and relevant clinical outcomes"; authors Luciano Pereira, Catarina Meng, Daniela Marques and João M. Frazão; Clinical Kidney Journal, 2018, vol 11, no.1, 80–88.

L. Pereira · J. M. Frazão (✉)
Institute of Investigation and Innovation in Health, University of Porto, Porto, Portugal

INEB – National Institute of Biomedical Engineering, University of Porto, Porto, Portugal

Department of Nephrology, São João Hospital Center, Porto, Portugal
e-mail: jmmdfrazao@gmail.com

L. Pereira
e-mail: lucianoarturpereira@hotmail.com

J. M. Frazão
DaVita Kidney Care, Amadora, Portugal

and inhibiting calcitriol synthesis and subsequently decreasing phosphate intestinal absorption. Also, the latter leads to a decreased gastrointestinal absorption of calcium with the subsequent development of hypocalcemia. The low calcitriol levels and hipocalcemia also stimulate PTH secretion in the parathyroid glands and induce the development of parathyroid gland hyperplasia and secondary hyperparathyroidism (SHPT).

Secondary hyperparathyroidism is associated with increased bone remodeling due to stimulation of the bone cells osteoblasts and osteoclasts. The result is the development of a high turnover bone disease called *osteitis fibrosa*. This bone disease is associated with increased risk of fractures, vascular calcifications, cardiovascular and all-cause mortality [4]. Recent observational data indicates that uncontrolled SHPT is associated with a higher risk of cardiovascular mortality as well as all-cause cardiovascular hospitalizations [5]. It is interesting to note that patients have better outcomes the longer the time they have controlled SPTH with intact PTH (iPTH) levels within the recommended range. Indeed consistent control of the bone metabolism parameters (iPTH, calcium and phosphate serum levels) within published recommended targets is a strong predictor of survival in hemodialysis patients [6].

The classical treatment for SHPT includes active vitamin D compounds and phosphate binders to limit gastrointestinal phosphate absorption [7]. However, achieving the optimal laboratory targets is often difficult because active vitamin D sterols have a small therapeutic window, suppressing PTH secretion, but simultaneously increasing calcium and phosphate intestinal absorption and serum levels.

Calcium sensing receptor (CaSR) is essential for maintaining systemic calcium homeostasis, becoming an excellent target for treating bone and mineral disorders. This receptor is expressed in several tissues including parathyroid gland cells [8]. Its ligands are called calcimimetics and can be classified as type 1 (agonists) such as ionized calcium and other divalent anions that directly stimulate CaSR or type 2 (positive allosteric modulators)—binding to a site that is distinct from the physiological ligand increasing the sensitivity of CaSR to ionized calcium, leading to the decrease of the set-point for systemic calcium homeostasis (homeostasis is achieved with lower concentrations of ionized calcium) [8]. This enables a decrease in plasma PTH levels, and consequently of calcium levels (Table 1). Additionally, lower levels of phosphorus and Calcium × Phosphorus are also seen [9], demonstrating the capability of calcimimetics to improve the four critical disease biomarkers associated with SHPT (phosphorus and calcium lowering effect distinguishes calcimimetics from active vitamin D) [10].

Table 1 Effect of PTH-suppressive therapies on biochemical parameters

	PTH	Calcium	Phosphorus	FGF-23
Vitamin D analogs	↓	↑	↑	↑
Cinacalcet	↓	↓	↓	↓
Etelcalcetide	↓↓	↓↓	↓	↓↓
Evocalcet	↓	↓	↓	↓

First generation compounds include phenylalkylamines R-567 and R-568 that were tested in hemodialysis patients but pharmacokinetics issues halted further clinical development [7]. Second generation calcimimetic drugs includes cinacalcet, and others never achieving clinical use such as calindol and AC-265347. Cinacalcet Hydrochloride was the first type 2 calcimimetic oral administered agent approved for clinical use [11].

Cinacalcet treatment effectively reduces PTH, calcium and phosphorus [12]. After more than 15 years from its approval, cinacalcet demonstrated that effectively reduces PTH and improves biochemical control of CKD-MBD.

Etelcalcetide is a new second generation calcimimetic. As a novel intravenous formulation with a pharmacokinetic profile that allows thrice-weekly dosing (at the time of hemodialysis), etelcalcetide was developed to improve efficacy and adherence and reduce gastrointestinal adverse effects relative to cinacalcet. It was recently approved in Europe and is regarded as a second opportunity to improve outcomes in CKD-MBD optimizing the treatment for SHPT using this promising new calcimimetic [13].

Evocalcet is the newly developed oral calcimimetic agent with less gastrointestinal adverse effects than cinacalcet and may be an alternative option for the treatment of secondary hyperparathyroidism in dialysis patients [14].

In this chapter, we summarize the impact of cinacalcet in biochemical and relevant clinical outcomes. We discuss the possible implications of etelcalcetide in the quest for improving outcomes for CKD patients. We also explore available data of the new oral calcimimetic evocalcet.

Cinacalcet Effectively Controls Secondary Hyperparathyroidism

Cinacalcet efficacy and safety was tested in several randomized controlled trials (RCTs) [11, 12, 15]. Cinacalcet treatment on addition to active vitamin D in patients with SHPT that are inadequately controlled despite standard therapy effectively decreases PTH levels along with reductions in serum calcium and phosphorus. Post hoc analysis demonstrated that treatment with cinacalcet improves achievement of biochemical targets recommended by international societies [16]. In a meta-analysis [17] involving 8 trials (1429 patients) comparing cinacalcet treatment plus standard therapy with placebo plus standard therapy end-of-treatment values for PTH (-290.49 pg/mL, 95% CI: -359.91 to -221.07), calcium (-0.85 mg/dL, 95% CI: -1.14 to -0.56), phosphorus (-0.29 mg/dL, 95% CI: -0.50 to -0.08) and calcium $\times$ phosphorus product (-7.90 mg^2/dL^2, 95% CI: -10.25 to -5.54) were significantly lower with cinacalcet compared with placebo.

To allow an objective assessment of the cinacalcet lowering effect of PTH, active vitamin D analogs dose was constant. However, subsequent clinical studies have confirmed the PTH-lowering effect of cinacalcet used in varying doses or constant doses of active vitamin D. This was an important finding considering that in clinical practice, cinacalcet is used often with vitamin D sterols [18]. Cinacalcet adverse effects are described in Table 2.

Besides the suppressive effect on PTH levels, data suggest that cinacalcet treatment can induce a volume reduction of the enlarged parathyroid glands with nodular hyperplasia seen in SHPT patients [19]. Meola et al. using high resolution color Doppler sonography measured parathyroid gland volume in nine hemodialysis patients with severe SHPT (mean baseline PTH 1196 ± 381 pg/mL) [20]. Patients were treated with cinacalcet, with a follow-up period of 24–30 months. Cinacalcet treatment led to a reduction in parathyroid gland volume in 68% in glands with a baseline volume < 500 mm^3 and in 54% in glands with a baseline volume ≥ 500 mm^3. In fact, cinacalcet exerts inhibitory effect on parathyroid cell proliferation in animal models of SPHT [21]. It is interesting to note that this inhibitory effect on cellular proliferation is specific for parathyroid cells and it is not observed in other cells expressing CaSR.

Table 2 Lateral effects of calcimimetic agents and suggested actions to take

Side effect	Frequency	Proposed action
Gastrointestinal events		
Nausea	Very common	Give Cinacalcet with main meal after dialysis/in the evening
Vomiting	Very common	
Diarrhea and dyspepsia	Uncommon	Decrease or fractionate the dose if symptoms appear after a dose increase
Anorexia	Common	Caution is advised with antiemetics, including metoclopramide (QT prolongation)
Hypocalcemia and nervous system disorders		
Hypocalcemia	Common	Withhold or reduce Cinacalcet until serum Calcium levels reach 8 mg/dl or symptoms have resolved
Dizziness and paraesthesia	Common	
Seizures	Uncommon	Use of Calcium-based phosphate binders, Vitamin D sterols or adjustments of dialysis fluid calcium have been suggested by some authors, according to clinical judgment
Others		
Skin and cutaneous disorders Rash	Common	Seek other causes. Consider discontinuing drug
Musculoskeletal, connective tissue and bone disorders Myalgia	Common	Seek other causes. Consider discontinuing drug
Immune-system disorders Hypersensitivity reactions	Uncommon	Seek other causes. Consider discontinuing drug

Cinacalcet Reduces FGF-23 Levels

FGF-23 levels have been associated with adverse clinical outcomes [22–27] progression of CKD, arterial calcification, left ventricle hypertrophy, cardiovascular events and increased mortality. A pharmacologic intervention capable of reducing FGF-23 holds the promise to have a beneficial effect on those important clinical outcomes.

CUPID (Cinacalcet Study for Peritoneal Dialysis Patients in Double Arm on the Lowing Effect of iPTH Level), a prospective, randomized controlled study, evaluated the effect of cinacalcet on FGF-23 levels [28] enrolled peritoneal dialysis patients for a period longer than 3 months and PTH > 300 pg/mL. Patients were randomized to cinacalcet therapy or vitamin D. Cinacalcet group had a reduction in FGF-23 levels (3960–2325 RU/mL) and the control group had an increase in FGF-23 concentration (2085–2415 RU/mL). ACHIEVE (ACHIEVE: Optimizing the Treatment of Secondary Hyperparathyroidism: A Comparison of Sensipar and Low Dose Vitamin D versus Escalating Doses of Vitamin D Alone), a phase 4, open-label, placebo-controlled, multicenter, RCT, was designed to compare treatment results with escalating doses of cinacalcet plus fixed low-dose calcitriol (cinacalcet-D group) versus escalating doses of calcitriol alone (Flex-D group) [29]. Using data of 91 subjects from this study, Wetmore et al. verified that the percentage change of FGF-23 between the two groups differed significantly (p = 0.002) [30]. In the Cinacalcet-D group the percentage change decreased (-9.7 ± 18.2; p = 0.021), while in the Flex-D group an increased tendency was found, however the results were not significant (4.1 ± 16.5).

The mechanism for this effect of cinacalcet on decreasing FGF-23 levels remains to be clarified. CUPID investigators concluded that cinacalcet treatment was independently associated with FGF-23 reduction, and not related with the drug's effect on PTH, calcium and phosphorus serum levels. Others observed that the decrease of FGF-23 levels is concomitant with the decrease in phosphorus levels (but not to PTH or calcium levels) [31]. Wetmore et al. suggested that calcium and phosphorus are responsible for cinacalcet's effect on FGF-23 levels [30]. Further investigation is needed in order to understand how exactly cinacalcet therapy results in greater reductions in serum FGF-23, when comparing to traditional drugs.

Recently, a post hoc evaluation of the EVOLVE (Evaluation of Cinacalcet Hydrochloride Therapy to Lower Cardiovascular Events) study added some more information to the FGF-23 issue [32]. When analyzing the results from the cinacalcet treated patients group (n = 1338) a decrease in FGF-23 levels was seen (5555–2255 pg/mL; p < 0.001), in opposition to the control group (n = 1264) where the levels remained unchanged (5600–5580 pg/mL). Moreover, when comparing to control group, a larger proportion of patients in the cinacalcet group had a meaningful decline ($\geq 30\%$) of FGF-23 (28% vs. 64%; p < 0.001). This finding is relevant, because the reduction $\geq 30\%$ of the FGF-23 levels was associated with a decreased risk of cardiovascular mortality (p < 0.001), sudden death (p < 0.001) and heart failure (p = 0.04).

Cinacalcet and Fractures

Patients with CKD have increased risk of fractures compared with the general population [33, 34]. Also there is a high rate of death and hospitalization following bone fracture among hemodialysis patients [35]. Abnormities in bone structure which affects bone quality are observed in patients with CKD-MBD. Malluche et al. demonstrated that bone with high turnover had material and nanomechanical abnormalities such as reduced mineral to matrix ratio [36]. The turnover-related alterations in bone quality may contribute to the diminished mechanical competence of bone in CKD.

Iimori et al. [37] in their single center cohort study demonstrated a U-shaped correlation between PTH and risk of fracture—only decreased [PTH < 150 pg/mL; Hazard ratio (HR) 3.27] or increased levels (PTH > 300 pg/mL; HR 2.69) were related to a superior hazard of clinical fracture.

There is no RCT specifically designed to evaluate whether any compound used in treatment of SHPT (phosphate binders, vitamin D analogs or calcimimetics) decreases the risk of fracture in CKD patients. However, treatment with cinacalcet has been associated with reduced risk of fractures. A combined post hoc analysis of safety data from four phase 3 RCTs enrolling 1184 patients with end-stage renal disease (ESRD) and uncontrolled SHPT (defined as PTH > 300 pg/mL) showed that randomization to cinacalcet on addition to conventional treatment with active vitamin D, resulted in significant reduction in the risk of fracture [Relative risk (RR) 0.46, 95% CI 0.22–0.95, p = 0.04] compared with placebo and conventional treatment [38].

In the EVOLVE trial, in the intention-to-treat (ITT) analysis cinacalcet did not significantly reduced the risk of fractures [39]. During the study, more than two thirds of patients in both groups discontinued the treatment, so a predetermined lag-censoring analysis (censoring time >6 months after stopping the study drug) was performed and a relative hazard for fracture of 0.72 (95% CI 0.58–0.90; p = 0.003) was obtained. When participants were censored at the time of co-interventions, such as parathyroidectomy and kidney transplant, the relative hazard was 0.71 (95% CI 0.58–0.87; p = 0.001). Moreover, when considering the risk of all clinical fractures (not only the first, but also the subsequent) the multivariable-adjusted relative hazard was 0.83 (95% CI 0.72–0.98; p = 0.02). Concluding, when taking into account events prompting discontinuation of the study drug, co-interventions and cumulative clinical fractures, cinacalcet reduced the rate of clinical fracture by 17–29% [39]. These data provide suggestive evidence that cinacalcet reduces risk of fracture in patients with SHPT.

This effect of cinacalcet in reducing fractures is not a surprising one considering two reports using bone histomorphometry from different groups describing improved histology in patients treated with cinacalcet [40, 41]. In BONAFIDE (Bone Biopsy Study for Dialysis Patients with Secondary Hyperparathyroidism of End Stage Renal Disease) [41] dialysis patients (n = 77) with PTH > 300 pg/mL and biopsy-proven high-turnover bone disease were treated with cinacalcet and a second bone biopsy was performed after 6–12 months of cinacalcet treatment. Bone formation and bone reabsorption indices were improved; most impressive was that the number of patients with normal bone histology increased from none at baseline from 20 to 12 months.

The role of bone mineral density (BMD) evaluation in chronic kidney patients is evolving. Unlike previous ones, current KDIGO guidelines suggest BMD testing in patients with CKD G3a-G5D with CKD-MBD and/or risk factors for osteoporosis if results will impact therapeutic decisions [42]. Evidence-based information is scarce about effect of cinacalcet on BMD in CKD patients. Some of available data showed a positive effect of cinacalcet on BMD, namely on femoral neck [43] and proximal femur [44]. However, others revealed that cinacalcet therapy showed no effect on BMD lumbar spine [44] or a detrimental effect with associated bone loss on femoral neck and lumbar spine [45]. The effect and significance of cinacalcet on BMD remains to be clarified.

Cinacalcet and Vascular Calcification

Secondary hyperparathyroidism is associated with vascular calcification. Once established in hemodialysis patients, it generally progresses much faster than in the general population, leading to an increased risk of all-cause and cardiovascular mortality [2].

In a single-center prospective cohort study (n=23), Nakayama et al. [46] evaluated the impact of cinacalcet in abdominal aortic calcification by calculating aortic calcification area index (ACAI) before and after treatment (−12, 0, 12, 24 and 36 months). The mean ACAI values were not decreased during the observation period (21.4% at baseline, 23.9% at 12 months, 23.7% at 24 months and 24.3% at 36 months). Tsuruta et al. [47] compared coronary artery calcification in a cinacalcet group (n=8) and a control group (n=60), verifying a decreasing tendency (−0.094/year) in the coronary artery calcification score when using cinacalcet, while in the control group the opposite was seen (+0.034/year). However, the results were not statistically significant (p=0.102).

ADVANCE (A Randomized Study to Evaluate the Effects of Cinacalcet Plus Low Dose Vitamin D on Vascular Calcification in Subjects with Chronic Kidney Disease) [48], compared vascular and cardiac valve calcification progression in 360 adult hemodialysis patients with SHPT, treated either with cinacalcet plus low-dose vitamin D (n=180) or flexible doses of vitamin D alone (n=180). The primary endpoint was changes in the Agatston Total Coronary Artery Calcification (CAC) score (uses the concept of plaque density, therefore reflecting the amount of calcium deposited within a calcified lesion). The median percent increase in Agatston total CAC score was not different between the two treatment groups. Similarly, Agatston Score changes in the thoracic aorta and mitral valve were not statistically significant. Aortic valve, on the other hand, had a stratified median treatment difference of −44.7% (95% CI: −85.8% to −6.1%; p=0.014).

The ADVANCE study had some limitations. A substantial number of patients assigned to cinacalcet group received doses of vitamin D higher than specified in protocol. A post hoc analysis [49] comparing CAC progression among protocol-adherent patients treated with cinacalcet showed that percentage increase in CAC and aortic valve calcification was significantly slower in cinacalcet group. Other limitations include the open-label design and short period of follow-up—12 months are unlikely to be sufficient to detect substantial changes in vascular calcification. Finally, the reduced observed calcification progression cannot be attributed solely to cinacalcet; we have to consider also the lower doses of vitamin D sterols in cinacalcet group.

Cinacalcet, Cardiovascular Disease and All-Cause Mortality

Elevated serum levels of phosphorus, calcium, PTH and FGF-23 have been linked to death and cardiovascular outcomes [50–52]. Cunningham et al. [38] in a post hoc analysis, combined data on clinical outcomes from four randomized phase 3, controlled trials and showed that treatment with cinacalcet resulted in a significant reduction in the risk of cardiovascular hospitalizations (HR = 0.61, 95% CI 0.43–0.86) and a non-significant tendency to reduce all-cause mortality. Another observational study including 19,186 hemodialysis patients from a large dialysis provider [53] receiving intravenous vitamin D analogs (as surrogate for the diagnosis of SHPT) found that the treatment with cinacalcet was associated with significant reductions in all-cause mortality, cardiovascular mortality, with more pronounced survival benefits founded in patients with more severe SHPT. In a prospectively observational study, Block et al. [50] described a significant survival benefit associated with cinacalcet prescription. These and others observations [54, 55] lead to the development of a prospective RCT evaluating the effect of cinacalcet treatment on cardiovascular mortality. The EVOLVE [56] was a RCT enrolling 3883 hemodialysis patients with moderate to severe SHPT (median PTH 693 pg/mL) assigned to receive cinacalcet (n = 1948) or placebo (n = 1935). All patients were eligible to receive conventional treatment including phosphate binders, vitamin D sterols. The primary composite end point was time until death, myocardial infarction, hospitalization for unstable angina, heart failure or a peripheral vascular event. In an unadjusted ITT analysis, the primary end point was reached in 48.2% of patients in cinacalcet group and 49.2% in placebo group (relative HR in the cinacalcet group 0.93; 95% CI 0.85–1.02; p = 0.11). After adjusting for baseline characteristics the relative HR for the primary composite end point was 0.88 (95% CI 0.79–0.97; p = 0.008). In fact, despite randomization there was an unexpected 1-year difference in age between groups (median age 55 years in cinacalcet group and 54 years in placebo group). As age is one of strongest predictions of death, this difference may have affected the results.

Also, the statistical power of EVOLVE was hampered by high rates of treatment crossover because discontinuation in the cinacalcet group (dropout) and use of commercially available cinacalcet in placebo group (drop-in). A pre-specified lag-censoring analysis in which data censored 6 months after patients stopped cinacalcet was performed. This analysis found a significant reduction in the risk of primary composite end point (HR 0.85; 95% CI 0.76–0.95; p = 0.003) and risk of death (HR 0.83; 95% CI 0.73–0.96; p = 0.009) in the cinacalcet group.

Another pre-determined protocol analysis compared younger (<65 years) and older patients (≥65 years) [57]. Cinacalcet reduced the risk of death and major CV events in older, but not younger patients.

Although the primary analysis of EVOLVE trial was negative, pre-specified additional analysis showed significant reduction in the risk of death or cardiovascular outcomes which suggests a potential benefit of cinacalcet.

Palmer et al. [58] published a metanalysis of randomized trials evaluating effects of calcimimetic therapy on mortality and adverse events in adults with CKD. Including 18 trials and a total of 7446 patients, they found cinacalcet had little or no effect on all-cause mortality (RR 0.97; 95% CI 0.89–1.05) and an imprecise effect on cardiovascular mortality (RR 0.67; 95% CI 0.16–2.87). The results of this metanalysis should be interpreted with caution. More than half of patients were derived from EVOLVE trial and this metanalysis only included the results from primary analysis with the potential setbacks that we discussed above. Also all trials included, except EVOLVE trial, were small and not specifically designed to assess clinical relevant outcomes such as mortality or cardiovascular events.

Etelcalcetide, A Novel Intravenous Calcimimetic Agent

Etelcalcetide is a novel second generation calcimimetic agent recently approved for the treatment of SHPT [13]. Etelcalcetide is a 8 amino acids peptide agonist of CaSR, which binds to CaSR by a covalente disulfide bond resulting in allosteric activation of CaSR and consequently reduced circulating levels of PTH and calcium [59]. In contrast to cinacalcet, etelcalcetide functions as a direct agonist of CaSR, slightly activating CaSR even under calcium-free conditions (Table 3). However, downstream signaling is stronger in the presence of calcium; thus the main action of etelcalcetide is mediated through its effects as allosteric activator [60].

Etelcalcetide has a favorable pharmacokinetic profile, with a longer elimination half-life than cinacalcet, with half-life elimination exceeding 7 days in ESRD patients [61]. It is administered by intravenous route at the end of hemodialysis session, with plasma concentration of etelcalcetide decreasing over time but remains relatively constant from 24 h post-dose to the next dialysis session [13]. It is a molecule dialysable during hemodialysis and with the doses of

Table 3 Comparison between cinacalcet and etelcalcetide. Values are expressed in percentage unless indicated otherwise. EAP: efficacy assessment phase

	Cinacalcet	Etelcalcetide
Class	Calcimimetic	Calcimimetic
Year of approval (Europe)	2004	2016
Mechanism of action	Interacts with membrane-spanning segments of CaSR and enhances signal transduction, thereby reducing PTH secretion	Peptide agonist of the CaSR that interacts with and activates the receptor thereby reducing PTH secretion
Mode of administration	Daily oral	IV at the end of dialysis
Half-life	30–40 h	>7 days
Excretion	Renal (80%), Fecal (15%)	Renal
Interaction with CYPs	Metabolized by CYP3A4, and to a lesser extent, CYP1A2; inhibits CYP2D6 (*caution is advised when prescribing potentially interacting drugs*)	No significant interactions
Daily dosing (starting; maximal)	30–180 mg	2.5–15 mg/dialysis
Efficacy endpoints >30% reduction from baseline in mean serum PTH level during the EAP >50% reduction from baseline in mean serum PTH during the EAP	63.9 40	77.9 52 (p = 0.001)
Adverse effects		
Nausea	22.6	18.3
Vomiting	13.8	13.3
Diarrhea	10.3	6.2
Headache	7.0	6.5
Hypertension	6.7	6.2
Hypotension	2.9	6.8
Muscle spasms	5.9	6.5
Pain in extremity	4.1	5.0
Asymptomatic hypocalcemia	59.8	68.9
Symptomatic hypocalcemia	2.3	5.0

etelcalcetide between 2.5 and 5 mg at the end of dialysis session, plasma concentrations of etelcalcetide reaches steady-state by week 4. Although clinical experience is of course limited, in vitro data shows data etelcalcetide is not an inhibitor, inducer or substrate of hepatic cytochrome (CYP) enzymes neither is an inhibitor or substrate of common efflux and uptake human transport proteins such as P-glycoprotein [62]. Thus, etelcalcetide is expected to have a low risk for CYP or transporter-mediated drug interactions.

Immunogenicity risk of etelcalcetide has been evaluated [63]. While both pre-existing and developing after treatment anti-etelcalcetide antibodies were detected, there are no consequences reported for clinical exposure, efficacy or safety of etelcalcetide.

Pivotal trials testing etelcalcetide in the treatment of SHPT were recently published [64, 65]. Two parallel, phase 3, placebo-controlled trials were conducted in 1023 hemodialysis patients with moderate to severe hyperparathyroidism. Intravenous administration of etelcalcetide (n = 503) or placebo (n = 513) after each hemodialysis session for 26 weeks was done. Patients randomized to etelcalcetide were significantly more likely to achieve primary efficacy end point (reduction greater than 30% in baseline PTH) 74.0–75.3% in etelcalcetide group versus 8.3–9.6% in placebo group. Also, patients randomized to etelcalcetide were significantly more likely to achieve a PTH level of 300 pg/mL or lower (49.6–53.3% in etelcalcetide group versus 4.6–5.1% in placebo group). The median dose of etelcalcetide during efficacy assessment phase was 5.0 and 7.1 mg. Patients randomized to etelcalcetide were more likely to experience substantial lowering of FGF-23 despite more frequent provision of calcium and vitamin D. Treatment with etelcalcetide decreased bone specific alkaline phosphatase and collagen type 1 cross-linked C-telopeptide. Patients randomized to etelcalcetide had more muscle spasms, nausea and vomiting than placebo group. Hypocalcemia occured in 63.8% of patients but symptomatic hypocalcemia was reported in only 7% of patients assigned to etelcalcetide. Similar results were obtained in a placebo-controlled trial from Japan, testing efficacy and safety of etelcalcetide [66].

A randomized, double-bind, double-dummy active clinical trial was conducted comparing intravenous etelcalcetide and oral placebo versus oral cinacalcet and intravenous placebo in 683 hemodialysis patients with PTH higher than 500 pg/mL [65]. The primary efficacy end point was non-inferiority of etelcalcetide at achieving more than a 30% reduction from baseline in mean predialysis PTH concentration and secondary end points included superiority in achieving biochemical end points (>50 and >30% reduction in PTH) and self-reported nausea or vomiting. Etelcalcetide was not inferior to cinacalcet in reducing PTH concentration and also met superior criteria. The proportion of patients who achieved >30% PTH reduction was 68.2% in etelcalcetide group and 57.7% in cinacalcet group. There was also a significant difference in proportions of patients who achieved >50% reduction of PTH. Hypocalcemia was more frequent in etelcalcetide group (68.9% vs. 59.8%) and the mean days of vomiting or nausea were not significantly different. Overall safety and tolerability between etelcalcetide and cinacalcet were similar. There was a numerically higher number of heart failure episodes in the etelcalcetide group, but overall the event rates were very low and similar to those observed in the EVOLVE trial.

The effect of etelcalcetide on FGF-23 levels is also noteworthy. Etelcalcetide treatment yielded more pronounced reduction in FGF-23 levels than cinacalcet. As discussed above, FGF-23 is elevated in CKD patients and it has been associated to adverse outcomes such as left ventricular hypertrophy and cardiac failure. Also in the EVOLVE trial a 30% reduction of FGF-23 levels was associated with significant reduction of primary composite end point, heart failure and death [32]. This promising finding in the etelcalcetide group raises the possibility of a more pronounced impact in cardiovascular outcomes.

There are some important clinical aspects to consider in the results of the referred trials we want to highlight. Etelcalcetide is superior to cinacalcet in achieving reduction of PTH and FGF-23 concentrations in ESRD patients, however also leading to more frequent episodes of hypocalcemia. Data suggests that this hypocalcemic effect could be more pronounced at beginning of treatment when PTH is highest. Indeed, in the multinational placebo-controlled trial, the calcium-lowering effect of etelcalcetide was evident early after treatment initiation and reached a nadir at weeks 10–12. This calcium-lowering effect was observed despite an increased use of oral calcium containing binders, active vitamin D analogs and increases in dialysate calcium concentration in an important proportion of patients. This observation might raise legitimate concerns regarding the possible cumulative positive calcium balance. Etelcalcetide is given at the end of hemodialysis session which improves medication adherence and reduces pill burden. Unlike previously anticipated, etelcalcetide does not seem to have fewer gastrointestinal symptoms related to calcimimetic treatment despite intravenous administration. The nausea and vomiting induced by cinacalcet and etelcalcetide appears to be a systemic effect rather than local gastrointestinal class effect.

Finally, it is tempting to consider that the longer elimination half-life could lead to a more stable control of biochemical parameters like PTH, calcium, phosphate and this sustained suppression of PTH could translate into improved bone turnover and metabolism, decreased vascular calcification and ultimately improved cardiovascular patient outcomes. This impact in such important outcomes remains to be proved.

Etelcalcetide—Questions to Resolve and (Some) Evidence from Outside the Clinical Trial World

There is still a paucity of published data of etelcalcetide in real world setting. However, there are some questions that remain to be answered and some emerging data that we want to highlight.

Etelcalcetide and Regression of Parathyroid Gland Size

Yoshimura et al. [67] reported a single case of dramatic reduction in parathyroid gland in a hemodialysis patient with uncontrolled SHPT in spite of treatment with active vitamin D and cicalcalcet. Oral cinacalcet was stopped and the patient was treated with etelcalcetide resulting in a decrease of total parathyroid glands volume from 1549 to 82.6 mm^3 after 9 months of treatment. Although this is an anecdotal report, it raises the hope that etelcalcetide can reduce the size of parathyroid gland even in patients who did not respond to cinacalcet. However, it remains to clarify if etelcalcetide induces apoptosis in hyperplastic parathyroid cells.

Etelcalcetide and Gastrointestinal Adverse Effects

Perhaps the most disappointing result of etelcalcetide pivotal trials was the absence of improved tolerance as it was anticipated considering the IV administration route. In the previously describe trial comparing cinacalcet with etelcalcetide, the adjusted mean weekly days of vomiting or nausea in the first 8 weeks of treatment were not significantly different for patients randomized to cinacalcet (0.3) and etelcalcetide (0.4) [65]. Of the 341 patients treated with cinacalcet, 77 (22.6%) reported nausea and 47 (13.8%) vomiting. Of the 338 patients randomized to etelcalcetide 62 (18.3%) reported nausea and 45 (13.3%) vomiting. Overall safety and tolerability between etelcalcetide and cinacalcet were similar.

In our personal clinical experience, etelcalcetide seems to perform better than cinacalcet regarding to nausea and vomiting. In future, further clinical evidence will confirm or refute this first clinical practice impression. In meantime, Mima et al. described 9 hemodialysis patients, with mean baseline PTH levels 626 ± 326 pg/mL, treated with etelcalcetide with an observation period of 4.4 ± 1.0 months [68]. The mean etelcalcetide dose was 6.1 ± 2.2 mg/hemodialysis session. Serum PTH levels decreased to 258 ± 207 pg/mL. In this very small study, no adverse events were reported during the observation period—nausea, vomiting, hypotension, headache, muscle spasms, anemia or abnormal 12-lead electrocardiograms.

Etelcalcetide and Theoretical Concerns of Its Use in Diabetics Undergoing Hemodialysis

There are some authors considering that until more clinical experience with etelcalcetide is available, the clinicians should be cautious when treating SHPT in diabetic hemodialysis patients with this new calcimimetic agent [69]. This is due to the theoretical possibility that etelcalcetide plasma protein binding may compete with oral hypoglycemic and insulins detemir and degludec, increasing the risk for hypoglycemia or hypocalcemia. Also hypocalcemia may cause decompensation of preexisting cardiac failure and lead to hypotension-related cardiac events, such as myocardial ischemia. Insulin-related hypoglycemia and hemodialysis prolong QT interval as well as hypocalcemia. So diabetic patients should be strictly monitored for hypocalcemia and associated effects.

Hypocalcemia in Hemodialysis Patients Treated with Calcimimetics

The 2009 KDIGO guidelines suggested in patients with CKD stages 3-5D to maintain serum calcium in normal range [2]. The revised 2017 KDIGO guidelines states that "in adult patients with CKD G3a-5D, we suggest avoiding hypercalcemia". The suggestion to avoid hypercalcemia is justified by novel evidence linking higher calcium levels to increased mortality in adults with CKD [42]. But there were doubts about the generalizability of the previous suggestion to correct hypocalcemia because of 2 arguments. First, there is the potential harm for some adults associated with positive calcium balance—it is important to remember that serum calcium levels do not necessarily reflect calcium balance [70, 71]. Second, the prevalence of hypocalcemia may have increased after introduction of cinacalcet [9, 72]. Most importantly, no negative signals were associated with the persistently low serum calcium levels in the cinacalcet arm of the EVOLVE trial [56]. So the clinical implications of hypocalcemia in the patients treated with calcimimetics is uncertain, but it may be less harmfull.

Floege J. et al. published an interesting work aiming to investigate incidence, predictors and therapeutic consequences of hypocalcemia by a post hoc analysis of EVOLVE [73]. At least one episode of hypocalcemia occurred within 16 weeks after the first administered dose of cinacalcet in 58.3% of patients compared to 14.9% of patients randomized to placebo. Hypocalcemia was severe (defined as total serum calcium < 7.5 mg/dL) in 18.4% in cinacalcet group compared with 4.4% in placebo group. In the majority of patients, hypocalcemia was asymptomatic and resolved spontaneously within 14 days with no modification of therapy. Among patients who received an intervention, the most common was an increase in active vitamin D dose. Interestingly, there were no increase in PTH following the hypocalcemia episode.

In summary, we agree with the KDIGO recommendation that is not necessary to correct hypocalcemia in all patients but significant or symptomatic hypocalcemia still should be addressed. Severe or symptomatic hypocalcemia could translate into adverse consequence such as bone disease, hyperparathyroidism and QT interval prolongation.

Evocalcet—A New Alternative Oral Calcimimetic Agent

Evocalcet is a newly synthesized oral calcimimetic agent [74]. In a rat model of renal failure, evocalcet and cinacalcet suppressed the secretion of PTH. However, cinacalcet induced a significant delay in gastric emptying while evocalcet did not. Evocalcet also induced less emesis compared with cinacalcet in common marmosets.

Recently a head-to-head comparison of efficacy and safety of evocalcet to cinacalcet was performed in Japanese hemodialysis patients with secondary hyperparathyroidism [14]. It was a phase 3, randomized double-blind, double-dummy trial. This study enrolled Japanese patients with SHPT that were randomized to evocalcet or cinacalcet for 30 weeks (317 patients each arm). The primary efficacy endpoint was non-inferiority of evocalcet to cinacalcet in the proportion of patients achieving a mean PTH level of 60–240 pg/mL. In the evocalcet arm, 72.7% of patients achieved PTH target compared with 76.7% of patients with cinacalcet group (between-group difference: −4% [confidence interval −11.4%; 3.5%], for non-inferiority). Gastrointestinal-related adverse effects occurred in 18.6% of patients treated with evocalcet and in 32.8% of patients treated with cinacalcet (between-group difference: −14.2% [−20.9%, −7.5%], significant for superiority). Other endpoints, serum calcium, serum phosphate, and FGF-23 decreased over time similarly in both groups.

Further studies are necessary to prove efficacy and safety of this new agent, namely in other populations and with different baseline and target PTH levels. We believe that evocalcet could be an interesting alternative to cinacalcet in hemodialysis, peritoneal dialysis patients, and possibly in other clinical contexts like primary hyperparathyroidism and parathyroid carcinoma.

Conclusion

In conclusion, SHPT is associated with increased bone turnover, risk of fractures, vascular calcifications, cardiovascular and all-cause mortality. Cinacalcet, the first calcimimetic approved for clinical use, effectively reduces PTH and improves biochemical control of mineral and bone disorders in chronic kidney patients. However, the effect of cinacalcet on hard outcomes remains to be proved.

Etelcalcetide, the new second generation calcimimetic, is superior to cinacalcet in achieving reduction of PTH and FGF-23 concentrations in ESRD patients. Also leads to more frequent episodes of hypocalcemia that could be more pronounced at beginning of treatment. Etelcalcetide is given at the end of hemodialysis session which improves medication adherence and reduces pill burden. Etelcalcetide has also unmet needs—besides hypocalcemia and unlike previously anticipated, etelcalcetide did not prove to have fewer gastrointestinal symptoms despite intravenous administration.

In our view, etelcalcetide represents significant advances in treatment of SHPT—better control of PTH, FGF-23, improved adherence. However if this improved biochemical control translates into improved clinical outcomes such as bone fractures rate, cardiovascular morbidity and mortality remains to be elucidated by prospective randomized trials.

Evocalcet is the new calcimimetic agent for the treatment of secondary hyperparathyroidism. In Japanese hemodialysis patients, this compound was better tolerated than cinacalcet.

Disclosure Luciano Pereira received speaker honoraria and travel grant from Amgen. João Frazão received consulting, speaker and travel honoraria from Amgen.

References

1. Jha V, Garcia-Garcia G, Iseki K, et al. Chronic kidney disease: global dimension and perspectives. Lancet. 2013;382(9888):260–72.
2. KDIGO clinical practice guideline for the diagnosis, evaluation, prevention, and treatment of Chronic Kidney Disease-Mineral and Bone Disorder (CKD-MBD). Kidney Int Suppl. 2009; (113):S1–130.
3. Diniz H, Frazao JM. The role of fibroblast growth factor 23 in chronic kidney disease-mineral and bone disorder. Nefrologia. 2013;33(6):835–44.
4. Kalantar-Zadeh K, Kuwae N, Regidor DL, et al. Survival predictability of time-varying indicators of bone disease in maintenance hemodialysis patients. Kidney Int. 2006;70(4):771–80.
5. Tentori F, Wang M, Bieber BA, et al. Recent changes in therapeutic approaches and association with outcomes among patients with secondary hyperparathyroidism on chronic hemodialysis: the DOPPS study. Clin J Am Soc Nephrol. 2015;10(1):98–109.
6. Danese MD, Belozeroff V, Smirnakis K, Rothman KJ. Consistent control of mineral and bone disorder in incident hemodialysis patients. Clin J Am Soc Nephrol. 2008;3(5):1423–9.
7. Rodriguez M, Goodman WG, Liakopoulos V, Messa P, Wiecek A, Cunningham J. The use of calcimimetics for the treatment of secondary hyperparathyroidism: a 10 year evidence review. Semin Dial. 2015;28(5):497–507.
8. Harrington PE, Fotsch C. Calcium sensing receptor activators: calcimimetics. Curr Med Chem. 2007;14(28):3027–34.
9. St Peter WL, Li Q, Liu J, et al. Cinacalcet use patterns and effect on laboratory values and other medications in a large dialysis organization, 2004 through 2006. Clin J Am Soc Nephrol. 2009;4(2):354–60.
10. Frazao J, Rodriguez M. Secondary hyperparathyroidism disease stabilization following calcimimetic therapy. NDT Plus. 2008;1(Suppl 1):i12–7.
11. Lindberg JS, Culleton B, Wong G, et al. Cinacalcet HCl, an oral calcimimetic agent for the treatment of secondary hyperparathyroidism in hemodialysis and peritoneal dialysis: a randomized, double-blind, multicenter study. J Am Soc Nephrol. 2005;16(3):800–7.
12. Block GA, Martin KJ, de Francisco AL, et al. Cinacalcet for secondary hyperparathyroidism in patients receiving hemodialysis. N Engl J Med. 2004;350(15):1516–25.
13. Blair HA. Etelcalcetide: First global approval. Drugs. 2016;76(18):1787–92.
14. Fukagawa M, Shimazaki R, Akisawa T, Evocalcet study group. Head to head comparison of the new calcimimetic agent evocalcet with cinacalcet in Japanese hemodialysis patients with secondary hyperparathyroidism. Kidney Int. 2018;94(4):818–25.
15. Goodman WG, Hladik GA, Turner SA, et al. The Calcimimetic agent AMG 073 lowers plasma parathyroid hormone levels in hemodialysis patients with secondary hyperparathyroidism. J Am Soc Nephrol. 2002;13(4):1017–24.
16. Moe SM, Chertow GM, Coburn JW, et al. Achieving NKF-K/DOQI bone metabolism and disease treatment goals with cinacalcet HCl. Kidney Int. 2005;67(2):760–71.
17. Strippoli GF, Palmer S, Tong A, Elder G, Messa P, Craiq JC. Meta-analysis of biochemical and patient-level effects of calcimimetic therapy. Am J Kidney Dis. 2005;47(5):715–26.
18. Stubbs JR, Wetmore JB. Does it matter how parathyroid hormone levels are suppressed in secondary hyperparathyroidism? Semin Dial. 2011;24(3):298–306.
19. Komaba H, Nakanishi S, Fujimori A, et al. Cinacalcet effectively reduces parathyroid hormone secretion and gland volume regardless of pretreatment gland size in patients with secondary hyperparathyroidism. Clin J Am Soc Nephrol. 2010;5(12):2305–14.
20. Meola M, Petrucci I, Barsotti G. Long-term treatment with cinacalcet and conventional therapy reduces parathyroid hyperplasia in severe secondary hyperparathyroidism. Nephrol Dial Transpl. 2009;24(3):982–9.
21. Olgaard K et al. The spectrum of mineral and bone disorders in chronic kidney disease, vol. 26. New York: Oxford University Press;2010. p. 443–58.

22. Isakova T, Xie H, Yang W, et al. Fibroblast growth factor 23 and risks of mortality and end-stage renal disease in patients with chronic kidney disease. JAMA. 2011;305(23):2432–9.

23. Fliser D, Kollerits B, Neyer U, et al. Fibroblast growth factor 23 (FGF23) predicts progression of chronic kidney disease: the Mild to Moderate Kidney Disease (MMKD) Study. J Am Soc Nephrol. 2007;18(9):2600–8.

24. Nasrallah MM, El-Shehaby AR, Salem MM, Osman NA, El Sheikh E, Sharaf El Din UA. Fibroblast growth factor-23 (FGF-23) is independently correlated to aortic calcification in haemodialysis patients. Nephrol Dial Transpl. 2010;25(8):2679–85.

25. Gutierrez OM, Januzzi JL, Isakova T, et al. Fibroblast growth factor 23 and left ventricular hypertrophy in chronic kidney disease. Circulation. 2009;119(19):2545–52.

26. Seiler S, Reichart B, Roth D, Seibert E, Fliser D, Heine GH. FGF-23 and future cardiovascular events in patients with chronic kidney disease before initiation of dialysis treatment. Nephrol Dial Transpl. 2010;25(12):3983–9.

27. Nakano C, Hamano T, Fujii N, et al. Intact fibroblast growth factor 23 levels predict incident cardiovascular event before but not after the start of dialysis. Bone. 2012;50(6):1266–74.

28. Kim HJ, Kim H, Shin N, et al. Cinacalcet lowering of serum fibroblast growth factor-23 concentration may be independent from serum Ca, P, PTH and dose of active vitamin D in peritoneal dialysis patients: a randomized controlled study. BMC Nephrol. 2013;14:112.

29. Fishbane S, Shapiro WB, Corry DB, et al. Cinacalcet HCl and concurrent low-dose vitamin D improves treatment of secondary hyperparathyroidism in dialysis patients compared with vitamin D alone: the ACHIEVE study results. Clin J Am Soc Nephrol. 2008;3(6):1718–25.

30. Wetmore JB, Liu S, Krebill R, Menard R, Quarles LD. Effects of cinacalcet and concurrent low-dose vitamin D on FGF23 levels in ESRD. Clin J Am Soc Nephrol. 2010;5(1):110–6.

31. Kuczera P, Adamczak M, Wiecek A. Cinacalcet treatment decreases plasma fibroblast growth factor 23 concentration in haemodialysed patients with chronic kidney disease and secondary hyperparathyroidism. Clin Endocrinol (Oxf). 2014;80(4):607–12.

32. Moe SM, Chertow GM, Parfrey PS, et al. Cinacalcet, fibroblast growth factor-23, and cardiovascular disease in hemodialysis: the evaluation of cinacalcet HCl therapy to lower cardiovascular events (EVOLVE) trial. Circulation. 2015;132(1):27–39.

33. Nickolas TL, McMahon DJ, Shane E. Relationship between moderate to severe kidney disease and hip fracture in the United States. J Am Soc Nephrol. 2006;17(11):3223–32.

34. Kaji H, Suzuki M, Yano S, et al. Risk factors for hip fracture in hemodialysis patients. Am J Nephrol. 2002;22(4):325–31.

35. Tentori F, McCullough K, Kilpatrick RD, et al. High rates of death and hospitalization following bone fracture among hemodialysis patients. Kidney Int. 2014;85(1):166–73.

36. Malluche HH, Porter DS, Monier-Faugere MC, Mawad H, Pienkowski D. Differences in bone quality in low- and high-turnover renal osteodystrophy. J Am Soc Nephrol. 2012;23(3):525–32.

37. Iimori S, Mori Y, Akita W, et al. Diagnostic usefulness of bone mineral density and biochemical markers of bone turnover in predicting fracture in CKD stage 5D patients—a single-center cohort study. Nephrol Dial Transpl. 2012;27(1):345–51.

38. Cunningham J, Danese M, Olson K, Klassen P, Chertow GM. Effects of the calcimimetic cinacalcet HCl on cardiovascular disease, fracture, and health-related quality of life in secondary hyperparathyroidism. Kidney Int. 2005;68(4):1793–800.

39. Moe SM, Abdalla S, Chertow GM, et al. Effects of cinacalcet on fracture events in patients receiving hemodialysis: the EVOLVE trial. J Am Soc Nephrol. 2015;26(6):1466–75.

40. Malluche HH, Monier-Faugere MC, Wang G, et al. An assessment of cinacalcet HCl effects on bone histology in dialysis patients with secondary hyperparathyroidism. Clin Nephrol. 2008;69(4):269–78.

41. Behets GJ, Spasovski G, Sterling LR, et al. Bone histomorphometry before and after long-term treatment with cinacalcet in dialysis patients with secondary hyperparathyroidism. Kidney Int. 2015;87(4):846–56.

42. Ketteler M, Block GA, Evenepoel P, et al. Executive summary of the 2017 KDIGO Chronic Kidney Disease-Mineral and Bone Disorder (CKD-MBD) guideline update: what's changed and why it matters. Kidney Int. 2017;92(1):26–36.
43. Tsuruta Y, Okano K, Kikuchi K, Tsuruta Y, Akiba T, Nitta K. Effects of cinacalcet on bone mineral density and bone markers in hemodialysis patients with secondary hyperparathyroidism. Clin Exp Nephrol. 2013;17:120–p126.
44. Lien YH, Silva AL, Whittman D. Effects of cinacalcet on bone mineral density in patients with secondary hyperparathyroidism. Nephrol Dial Transpl. 2005;20:1232–7.
45. Mitsopoulos E, Ginikopoulou E, Economidou D, et al. Impact of long-term cinacalcet, ibandronate or teriparatide therapy on bone mineral density of hemodialysis patients: a pilot study. Am J Nephrol. 2012;36:238–44.
46. Nakayama K, Nakao K, Takatori Y, et al. Long-term effect of cinacalcet hydrochloride on abdominal aortic calcification in patients on hemodialysis with secondary hyperparathyroidism. Int J Nephrol Renovasc Dis. 2013;7:25–33.
47. Tsuruta Y, Ohbayashi T, Fujii M, et al. Change in coronary artery calcification score due to cinacalcet hydrochloride administration. Ther Apher Dial. 2008;12(Suppl 1):S34–7.
48. Raggi P, Chertow GM, Torres PU, et al. The ADVANCE study: a randomized study to evaluate the effects of cinacalcet plus low-dose vitamin D on vascular calcification in patients on hemodialysis. Nephrol Dial Transpl. 2011;26(4):1327–39.
49. Urena-Torres PA, Floege J, Hawley CM, et al. Protocol adherence and the progression of cardiovascular calcification in the ADVANCE study. Nephrol Dial Transpl. 2013;28(1):146–52.
50. Block GA, Klassen PS, Lazarus JM, Ofsthun N, Lowrie EG, Chertow GM. Mineral metabolism, mortality, and morbidity in maintenance hemodialysis. J Am Soc Nephrol. 2004;15(8):2208–18.
51. Floege J, Kim J, Ireland E, et al. Serum iPTH, calcium and phosphate, and the risk of mortality in a European haemodialysis population. Nephrol Dial Transpl. 2011;26(6):1948–55.
52. Gutierrez OM, Mannstadt M, Isakova T, et al. Fibroblast growth factor 23 and mortality among patients undergoing hemodialysis. N Engl J Med. 2008;359(6):584–92.
53. Block GA, Zaun D, Smits G, et al. Cinacalcet hydrochloride treatment significantly improves all-cause and cardiovascular survival in a large cohort of hemodialysis patients. Kidney Int. 2010;78(6):578–89.
54. Akizawa T, Kurita N, Mizobuchi M, et al. PTH-dependence of the effectiveness of cinacalcet in hemodialysis patients with secondary hyperparathyroidism. Sci Rep. 2016;6:19612.
55. Gillespie IA, Floege J, Gioni I, et al. Propensity score matching and persistence correction to reduce bias in comparative effectiveness: the effect of cinacalcet use on all-cause mortality. Pharmacoepidemiol Drug Saf. 2015;24(7):738–47.
56. Chertow GM, Block GA, Correa-Rotter R, et al. Effect of cinacalcet on cardiovascular disease in patients undergoing dialysis. N Engl J Med. 2012;367(26):2482–94.
57. Parfrey PS, Drueke TB, Block GA, et al. The Effects of cinacalcet in older and younger patients on hemodialysis: the evaluation of cinacalcet HCl therapy to lower cardiovascular events (EVOLVE) trial. Clin J Am Soc Nephrol. 2015;10(5):791–9.
58. Palmer SC, Nistor I, Craig JC, et al. Cinacalcet in patients with chronic kidney disease: a cumulative meta-analysis of randomized controlled trials. PLoS Med. 2013;10(4):e1001436.
59. Alexander ST, Hunter T, Walter S, et al. Critical cysteine residues in both the calcium-sensing receptor and the allosteric activator AMG 416 underlie the mechanism of action. Mol Pharmacol. 2015;88(5):853–65.
60. Walter S, Baruch A, Dong J, et al. Pharmacology of AMG 416 (Velcalcetide), a novel peptide agonist of the calcium-sensing receptor, for the treatment of secondary hyperparathyroidism in hemodialysis patients. J Pharmacol Exp Ther. 2013;346(2):229–40.

61. Chen P, Melhem M, Xiao J, Kuchimanchi M, Perez Ruixo JJ. Population pharmacokinetics analysis of AMG 416, an allosteric activator of the calcium-sensing receptor, in subjects with secondary hyperparathyroidism receiving hemodialysis. J Clin Pharmacol. 2015;55(6):620–8.
62. Subramanian R, Zhu X, Kerr SJ, et al. Nonclinical pharmacokinetics, disposition, and drug-drug interaction potential of a novel d-amino acid peptide agonist of the calcium-sensing receptor AMG 416 (Etelcalcetide). Drug Metab Dispos. 2016;44(8):1319–31.
63. Kroenke MA, Weeraratne DK, Deng H, et al. Clinical immunogenicity of the d-amino acid peptide therapeutic etelcalcetide: Method development challenges and anti-drug antibody clinical impact assessments. J Immunol Methods. 2017;445:37–44.
64. Block GA, Bushinsky DA, Cunningham J, et al. Effect of etelcalcetide vs placebo on serum parathyroid hormone in patients receiving hemodialysis with secondary hyperparathyroidism: two randomized clinical trials. JAMA. 2017;317(2):146–55.
65. Block GA, Bushinsky DA, Cheng S, et al. Effect of etelcalcetide vs cinacalcet on serum parathyroid hormone in patients receiving hemodialysis with secondary hyperparathyroidism: a randomized clinical trial. JAMA. 2017;317(2):156–64.
66. Fukagawa M, Yokoyama K, Shigematsu T, et al. A phase 3, multicentre, randomized, double-blind, placebo-controlled, parallel-group study to evaluate the efficacy and safety of etelcalcetide (ONO-5163/AMG 416), a novel intravenous calcimimetic, for secondary hyperparathyroidism in Japanese haemodialysis patients. Nephrol Dial Transpl. 2017;10:1723–30.
67. Yoshimura K, Funakoshi Y, Terawaki H. Dramatic regression of parathyroid gland swelling after conversion of calcimimetic medication from cinacalcet to etelcalcetide. Ther Apher Dial. 2018;22(5):553–4.
68. Mima A, Tansho K, Nagahara D, Watase K. Treatment of secondary hyperparathyroidism in patients on hemodialysis using a novel synthetic peptide calcimimetic, etelcalcetide: a short-term clinical study. J Int Med Res. 2018;46(11):4578–85.
69. Ye J, Deng G, Gao F. Theoretical overview of clinical and pharmacological aspects of the use of etelcalcetide in diabetic patients undergoing hemodialysis. Drug Des Devel Ther. 2018;12:901–9.
70. Raggi P, Bommer J, Chertow GM. Valvular calcification in hemodialysis patients randomized to calcium-based phosphorus binders or sevelamer. J Heart Valve Dis. 2004;13:134–41.
71. Spiegel DM, Brady K. Calcium balance in normal individuals and in patients with chronic kidney disease on low- and high-calcium diets. Kidney Int. 2012;81:1116–21.
72. Chonchol M, Locatelli F, Abboud HE, et al. A randomized double-blind, placebo-controlled study to assess the efficacy and safety of cinacalcet HCl in participants with CKD not receiving dialysis. Am J Kid Dis. 2009;53:197–207.
73. Floege J, et al. Incidence, predictors and therapeutic consequences of hypocalcemia in patients treated with cinacalcet in the EVOLVE trial. Kidney Int. 2018;93(6):1475–82.
74. Kawata T, et al. A novel calcimimetic agent, evocalcet (MT-4580/KHK7580) suppresses the parathyroid cell function with litlle effect on the gastrointestinal tract or CYP isozymes in vivo and in vitro. PLoS ONE. 2018;13(4):e0195316.

Parathyroidectomy in Chronic Kidney Disease

Sandro Mazzaferro, Silverio Rotondi, Martia Pasquali, Angelo
Mazzarella and Lida Tartaglione

Definition and Pathogenesis of CKD-MBD

Chronic Kidney Disease (CKD) with the eventual Chronic Renal Failure (CRF) associates with a maladaptive response in the homeostasis of mineral metabolism, characterized by modifications in serum level not only of calcium and phosphate but also of old and new hormones now recognized to be linked with worse clinical outcomes [1]. Hormones particularly involved with homeostasis and side effects are: Parathyroid hormone (PTH), 1,25-dihydroxyvitamin D and the recently described fibroblast growth-factor 23 (FGF23) with its important co-receptor, Klotho. PTH and vitamin D are the two old fashioned mineral metabolism hormones; for long time they have been considered the exclusive playing actors in the pathogenesis of secondary hyperparathyroidism (SHPT) of CKD [2]. It was believed that, in renal patients, an increment in serum phosphate reduced circulating levels of calcium which was responsible for increased synthesis and secretion of PTH leading to parathyroid cells hypertrophy and, in the long term, hyperplasia. This secondary raise in PTH secretion was meant to restore the physiologic calcium-phosphate homeostasis by increasing renal phosphate excretion and calcium reabsorption. However, subsequent observations evidenced that in the very early stages of CKD serum calcium levels are still in the normal range but serum phosphate are possibly reduced, which challenged such hypothesis. Since the early "hypophosphatemic" stage associated with reduced levels of the

S. Mazzaferro (✉) · S. Rotondi · M. Pasquali · A. Mazzarella · L. Tartaglione
Department of Translational and Precision Medicine, Sapienza University of Rome, Rome,
Italy
e-mail: Sandro.mazzaferro@uniroma1.it

S. Mazzaferro · S. Rotondi · M. Pasquali · A. Mazzarella · L. Tartaglione
Policlinico Umberto I Hospital, Nephrology Unit, Rome, Italy

© Springer Nature Switzerland AG 2020
A. Covic et al. (eds.), *Parathyroid Glands in Chronic Kidney Disease*,
https://doi.org/10.1007/978-3-030-43769-5_12

active vitamin D metabolite (explained by impaired 1-alpha-hydroxylation activity in the damaged tubular cells), hypocalcemia could be regarded as secondary to vitamin D deficiency. Further, the discovery of calcium and vitamin D receptors (CaSR and VDR) and the evidence that their tissue expression is reduced in uremic patients allowed to introduce new pathogenetic mechanisms of SHPT: the resistance of uremic tissues to PTH and the left-shifting of the calcium set point in the calcium-PTH response curve [3]. However, even these findings still not satisfied the complexity of the variable biochemical and clinical picture of SHPT. Recently, new pathogenetic hypotheses are consented by the discovery of FGF23 and Klotho. FGF23, definitely a new player in the field of SHPT, [4] is a phosphatonin produced by osteoblasts that regulates phosphate and vitamin D balance by increasing phosphaturia and by inhibiting renal 1-alpha-hydroxylase and vitamin D activation. Klotho, its co-receptor, is predominantly produced in the kidney and is essential for the renal selective effects of FGF23. It is thus possible that an early reduction of Klotho synthesis by the damaged kidney stimulates bone synthesis of FGF23 to overcome this "renal resistance" (Fig. 1, bottom panel). The increment of FGF23 could explain phosphaturia and lower active vitamin D synthesis. Intriguingly, both FGF23 and Klotho are also acknowledged of extra-renal and extra-bone effects that could be relevant for the systemic clinical picture of SHPT [5]. In fact, FGF23 is capable of direct myocardial effects which favor cardiac hypertrophy and of pro-inflammatory and immunosuppressive effects that may foster systemic inflammation [6]. As for Klotho, a circulating soluble fraction (sKlotho) is considered responsible for direct (FGF23-independent) biologic effects that are relevant to blunt the natural phenomenon of aging and the associated osteoporosis and vascular calcification [7]. In fact, the klotho null animal is considered an experimental model of accelerated aging. Conceivably, in early renal failure but also in non-renal subjects an excessive dietary phosphate load, with or without increments in serum phosphate levels, could stimulate FGF23 bone synthesis (through phosphate receptor in bone cells?) with the eventual changes in phosphate and vitamin D. Later, PTH will predictably increase. Notably, PTH and FGF23 exert opposite effects on vitamin D synthesis, since PTH stimulates whereas FGF23 inhibits renal hydroxylation of vitamin D. Vitamin D therapy, commonly employed in renal patients to reduce PTH hypersecretion, further stimulates FGF23 synthesis thus contributing to the very high levels of FGF23 typical of overt renal insufficiency. Indeed, FGF23 production by osteoblasts and osteocytes increases progressively along with renal function reduction probably due to the phosphate load faced by the residual single nephrons which supposedly have a threshold phosphate load over which tubular damage is produced. High levels of FGF23, phosphate and PTH and low levels of Klotho, vitamin D and calcium, typically encountered in renal insufficiency, are all associated with increased rate of morbidity and mortality. In summary, the intricacy of divalent ions homeostasis in CKD has definitely increased in recent years. SHPT now includes not only the biochemical modifications of divalent ions and of the related hormones but also the different pictures of renal bone disease (high turnover, low turnover or osteomalacia) and the associated acceleration of vascular

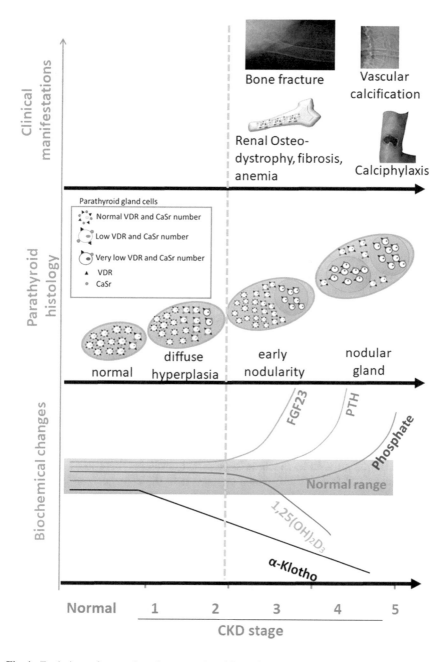

Fig. 1 Evolution of secondary hyperparathyroidism from biochemical changes in mineral metabolism (bottom panel), to histologic modifications of parathyroid cells (middle panel), to clinical manifestations (upper panel). VDR: Vitamin D receptors; CaSR: Calcium sensing receptors; FGF23: Fibroblast growth factor 23; PTH: Parathyroid hormone; 1,25(OH)2D3: 1,25 dihydroxy vitamin D; CRF: Chronic renal failure; CKD: Chronic Kidney disease

and ectopic calcifications. This ensemble carries the burden of systemic negative effects considered responsible, at least in part, of the increased all-cause and cardiovascular risk of these patients. Conceivably, SHPT represents a true clinical syndrome named CKD-MBD [8]. Also, CKD-MBD could be regarded as a model of accelerated aging helpful to discover new pathomechanisms and therapies for the general population [9]. Conceptually, the hormonal machinery that regulates divalent ions and maintains serum levels of calcium and phosphate within narrow ranges, becomes maladaptive and responsible for secondary organ damage when chronically and/or excessively activated either in normal subjects or in renal patients [1].

Modifications of Parathyroid Glands in CRF

In the presence of prolonged chronic stimulation of parathyroid hormone synthesis and secretion, as observed in CRF, we find histologic modifications of the parathyroid glands characterized by an initial simple hypertrophy that progressively changes into a polyclonal hyperplasia with an increase of the volume and number of cells in the glands. (Fig. 1, middle panel). This morphologic modification obviously involves all glands (orthotopic and ectopic). We may consider four different types of parathyroid hyperplasia [10]: diffuse hyperplastic gland, early nodularity in diffuse hyperplastic gland, nodular hyperplastic gland and single nodular gland. These pathologic aspects are characterized by a progressive increase in the number of oxyphil cells that progressively prevail in number the typical chief parathyroid cells. In this way the gland develops an increasing number of diffuse nodularity with the appearance of single parathyroid cell clones that synthesize and secrete amounts of parathyroid hormone independently of the resulting levels of serum calcium. Importantly, in as much as hyperplasia develops, there is a reduction of expression of CaSR and VDR, which explains how the cells become less responsive or non-responsive at all to the circulating levels of serum calcium and vitamin D. Currently, the histologic pattern of diffuse hyperplasia is considered sensitive to therapies (calcium supplements and vitamin D to increase serum levels of calcium, and/or vitamin D and calcimimetic to stimulate VDR and CaSR), while the nodular lesion is not and is typically characterized by overt hypercalcemia associated with persistently elevated PTH levels in the clinical setting of tertiary hyperparathyroidism [11]. In summary, SHPT develops progressively, and progressively becomes less responsive or non-responsive to the available medical therapies. Regrettably, persistently elevated PTH levels (ten to hundred times higher than upper normal values) severely damage bones which develop the high turnover— osteitis fibrosa lesion, responsible for pain, fractures and deformities that significantly reduce the quality of life and life expectancy of the affected patients. Also, hyperparathyroidism, especially if associated with high levels of serum calcium and phosphate definitely favours vascular and ectopic calcifications which are implicated in the increased cardiovascular burden of renal patients. As a whole, severe SHPT is a risky clinical condition with dishabilitating side effects (Fig. 1, upper panel), requiring prompt treatment. If medical therapy is ineffective, parathyroid surgery becomes necessary.

Indication, Rates and Types of Parathyroidectomy (PTX)

The international KDIGO Guidelines recommend PTX whenever a patient has severe and/or progressive SHPT that fails to respond to available medical therapies [12]. Indeed, despite growing pharmaceutical armamentarium a number of patients become unresponsive to drugs and PTX is unavoidable in some cases. In dialysis patients the prevalence of PTX increases along with the time spent on replacement therapy, and has been reported in about 15% after 10 years and 28% after 20 years of haemodialysis [13]. It is interesting to notice that the indication to PTX shows different trends along the time [14]. For example, in 2005 Foley recorded a significant drop in the incident rate of PTX (11.6 per 1000 patient-years in 1992 and 6.8 per 1000 patient-years in 1998) possibly coincident with the introduction in clinical practice of the intravenous formulation of calcitriol or to the wider availability of the intact PTH assay, less affected by inactive PTH fragments. Intriguingly, in the same study a rise in PTX was observed starting from 1998 and up to 2002 which could be referred to an increased attention not only to serum levels of PTH, but also to serum calcium and phosphate and to the risk of low turnover bone and ectopic calcifications with more aggressive and prolonged medical therapies. Also, the publication of the KDOQI (Kidney Disease Outcomes Quality Initiative) guidelines with specific reference ranges for calcium, phosphate and PTH [15], could have induced a less aggressive medical therapy and the eventual rise in PTX. Following to the KDOQI, also the KDIGO (Kidney Disease Improving Global Outcome) guidelines were published with an update of the reference range for serum PTH levels from 150–300 pg/ml to 2–9 times the upper limit of normality [16]. The effect of this change, together with the description of the existence of significant regional differences in the management of SHPT, are described in a study by Tentori et al. [17] This study examined the huge database of the DOPPS (Dialysis Outcomes and Practice Patterns Study) which is realized by a periodic and regular collection of biochemical and clinical outcomes of dialysis patients from countries all over the world. The report on SHPT by Tentori et al. included a first observation period, consisting of four different phases (DOPPS phases 1–4) from 1996 to 2011 and a total of 35.655 patients followed for a median of 1.6 years, and a second period consisting of the fifth DOPPS phase, from 2012 to 2015, which included 8.164 patients. Results were examined separately for the major countries involved (Europe, Australia-New Zealand, Japan and North America) and described the temporal trend of the average PTH values. Interestingly, from 1996 to 2008 (DOPPS phases 1–5), a significant increase of median values of PTH was observed in Australia-New Zealand, North America and Europe, at variance with no increment in Japan, in which country the number of patients at target increased. Since these results ante-dated the introduction of the KDIGO, they could not be related to changes in the PTH reference range (from 150–300 to 2–9 times the upper limit of normality), rather they testified the existence of different policies by different professional organizations. In fact, definitely lower values of PTH are recommended in Japan (60–180 pg/ml in 2008 and 60–240 in 2012). Importantly, the rising of PTH levels in Europe, Australia-New Zealand and North America was independent of serum levels of calcium (same trend in cases with values higher or lower than 9.2 mg/dl) or phosphate (same trend in cases with values higher or lower than 5.2 mg/dl) and of age or time spent on dialysis. Coincidentally, with these shifts in PTH levels, the study describes a significant reduction in the rate of PTX. Indeed, in a database including roughly 300.000 dialysis patients showing a PTX prevalence of 1.5%, significant geographic variations in the utilization of PTX have been reported also within the US regions only [18]. Finally, in a recent study includ-ing more than 30.000 PTX carried out in the US, a drop in PTX rates is reported, starting from 2004–2005 and possibly coincident with the introduction of the cal-cimimetic Cinacalcet [19]. In summary, the indication to PTX is not standardized but remains a therapeutic option for a minority but significant number of patients. Also, while it is not possible to address causality from observational studies like those available, it is evident that whenever new guidelines, therapies or biomarkers are offered clinicians modify their policy to indicate surgery.

When indicated, the surgical technique for PTX can be total, subtotal or total plus auto-transplantation. In general, the surgeon should search for all glands since all are presumably hyperplastic and surgery should be as definitive as possible given the increased risk of significant side effects (e.g. laryngeal paralysis) in case of neck re-operation. Total PTX, i.e. removal of all localized glands, is preferred by some surgeons, but not by nephrologists who fear the resulting hypoparathy-roidism and the associated condition of low PTH levels, adynamic bone disease and hypocalcemia. For this reason, subtotal PTX is the preferred technique, with removal of all localized glands except for 1/3rd of the smallest identified gland. Total PTX with auto transplantation is obtained by removal of all identified glands and reimplantation, in the forearm or other anatomic sites, of small fragments of parathyroid tissue selected from the best-preserved gland. The risks with this tech-nique are the autonomous proliferation and dissemination of the implanted tissue or the failure of implantation with resulting hypoparathyroidism. Observational data suggest that subtotal PTX and total PTX with auto transplantation have sim-ilar outcomes in terms of complications, readmission and 30-day mortality rate [20] or that Total PTX carries a lower risk of recurrence as compared to Total PTX plus auto transplantation [21] or that Total PTX plus auto transplantation and Subtotal PTX are similarly effective in terms of recurrence, persistence or reop-eration [22]. Again, there is no firm evidence of the superiority of one technique over others, thus evidencing that patient's selection and optimal surgical technique could represent a challenging issue for the practical nephrologist [23] In a recent multicentre observational study in Italy we reported that subtotal PTX was the most frequent type of surgery (55.0%), followed by total PTX (38.7%) and total PTX plus auto transplantation (6.3%) [24].

Clinical outcomes after PTX: Control of divalent ions

In the study by Tentori et al., [17] patients with PTH values higher than 300 pg/ml had an increased risk of all-cause and cardiovascular mortality and an increased hospitalization rate, while those with values lower than 50 pg/ml had an increased all-cause mortality rate. These findings are in agreement with a number of studies reporting on the association between too high or too low PTH values and morbidity or mortality. Similar findings are available for serum calcium and phosphate. Accordingly, the main target of clinicians recommending PTX should be to improve the biochemical control of SHPT. In our experience we observed, in a relatively small number of subjects followed up immediately after surgery and after one month and one, three and five years, that the prevalence of patients targeting serum calcium, phosphate or PTH may not be satisfactory [25]. Indeed, the prevalence of cases at target for PTH was less than 10% after 1, 3 and 5 years of follow-up, with a majority of cases with low values (<150 pg/ml). The best improvement was evident for serum phosphate with 65–76% of cases at target, while cases at target for serum calcium ranged between 37 and 15%, with a suggestive trend toward worsening along with the increment of follow-up. Another retrospective cohort study compared the same biochemical parameters one year before and one year after parathyroidectomy in 1402 dialysis patients [26]. PTH values, which showed a tendency to increase in the year before surgery, (from 1039 to 1661 pg/ml) dramatically dropped after glands removal to a low median values of 98 pg/ml (range 28–366 pg/ml) and there were still cases with too high values (10% showed PTH levels ≥ 897 pg/ml), thus confirming that PTX may be ineffective in targeting PTH values. In our recent multicentre study in Italy, prevalent parathyroidectomized patients represented roughly 4% of the dialysis population, were characterized by low PTH (<150 pg/ml) in 62% of the cases, and had serum levels of calcium or phosphate out of the range in 50% [24].

We can thus conclude that while PTX improves the control of very high (and dangerous) levels of PTH, it is not a guarantee of optimal biochemical control.

Clinical outcomes after PTX: Mortality and morbidity

Severe SHPT contributes to vessel wall calcification and cardiovascular and all-cause mortality in haemodialysis patients. Also, the damage of bone structure increases the risk and rate of fracture that further contribute to mortality. Accordingly, we could consider that the abovementioned biochemical targets are non-hard outcome parameters and that hard-clinical outcomes like mortality and/ or fractures should be regarded as more relevant. Indeed, the study by Foley [14] also analysed the risk of death following PTX in the two time intervals considered (94–95 and 98–99) and found an increased risk of death in the two months early after surgery which was followed, however, by a significant improvement in the following 6–12 months, which was then maintained for 5 years. Similarly, an increased mortality rate soon after surgery (in the early 3 months) has been reported also in another study in 4558 haemodialysis patients. While we could most probably relate this increment to increased surgical risk in these highly comorbid patients, the confirmed significant reduction of mortality rate in the long term could be surprising [27]. Data from the USRDS (United States Renal Database System) considering the event rates one year before and one year after PTX, also describes an increased rate of all cause hospitalization following surgery, to be mostly referred to episodes of hypocalcaemia in the 30 days after discharge thus underlying an increased morbidity early after surgery [28]. Another experience, from the Swedish Renal registry data, included 423 dialysis patients and 156 renal transplant patients who received PTX and a control group of non-PTX patients matched for age, sex and renal disease [29]. In this study, the reduction of mortality rate was demonstrated in dialysis cases only, suggesting that the two populations (dialysis and transplantation) with completely different biochemical and clinical conditions, may differently benefit from the same surgical therapy. The largest case-control study dealing with all-cause and cardiovascular mortality in parathyroidectomized dialysis patients comes from the Japan registry and includes 4,428 patients who received PTX and 4,428 propensity score matched cases who did not [30]. In the 1-year-follow-up period considered, PTX cases had a lower risk of mortality from both all-cause (4.3 vs. 6.5%) and CV disease (1.8 vs. 3.1%). Causes of death that were significantly different were heart failure, infection disease and cardiac arrest, which points to the role of PTH on cardiovascular and immunologic response. Also, crude, case mix or multivariate adjusted analysis confirmed, in patients who did not receive PTX, that either too low or too high PTH levels associate with increased risk of mortality. Although this study represents the strongest available evidence of the clinical advantage of PTX, it is still a retrospective, observational study with potential selection biases. However, as outlined in a commentary to this study, a prospective, randomized, and controlled clinical trial on PTX aiming at demonstrating that surgery is better than medical therapy, most probably will never be realized due to practical, economic and possibly ethical implications [31]. In the meanwhile, observational studies continue to be published, like the recent one reporting on the helpful role of improved surgical technique and of watchful post-PTX care on the improvement of survival [32].

Another hard outcome to consider in PTX patients is the risk of fracture. Rudser et al. compared incident hip, vertebral, and distal radius-wrist fractures between 6.000 PTX patients and 16.000 control and found lower cumulative incidence in PTX (32% lower risk for hip fracture and 31% for any analysed fracture) [33]. This finding is confirmed in a more recent publication including dialysis and transplanted patients (579 cases and 1970 matched controls) showing lower hip fracture risk in PTX (HR = 0.40, CI 0.18-0.88). However, after adjusting for sex and renal replacement therapy, the difference was not confirmed in males and in renal transplant patients [34]. Indeed, the role of PTX in the outcome of renal transplant patients is still unclear and should include also the outcome of the graft, and not of the patient only. Recent data suggest that patients with inadequate PTH control one-year post transplant should be better referred to the surgeon [35].

Regrettably, bone biopsy studies describing the effects of PTX on bone and that could be helpful to understand differences in outcome, are scanty. Hernandes et al. evaluated bone biopsy in 19 haemodialysis patients before and one year after PTX and described a substantial modification of histology which changed from osteitis fibrosa to adynamic bone in the majority of the cases. This study also evaluated coronary artery calcium score and suggested that the one-year increment of the calcification score was significantly associated with the development of low bone turnover [36]. In summary, although of limited methodologic reliability, all of the available data suggest that PTX associates with improved survival in the long term, even though an increment is possible immediately after surgery. This improvement has no firm clinical explanation, but could be related to the beneficial systemic effects potentially associated with the control of severe secondary hyperparathyroidism and that have been referred to the negative systemic effects of PTH (e.g. on heart, bone marrow, etc.).

Conclusion

In conclusion, PTX is still necessary in a limited but significant number of renal failure patients. Significant regional differences are evident, that clearly underline the absence of unequivocal guidelines. Surgical techniques are similarly effective, but subtotal PTX and total PTX plus auto transplantation are the two most frequently employed. PTX should not be regarded as essential to target biochemical targets of SHPT, rather it should be considered helpful to avoid the severity of SHPT which could carry clinical improvements in the long-term. Some increment in morbidity and mortality in the early period following surgery is predictable, but in the long term an improvement of survival is most often predictable. As a whole, it seems that nephrologists do not still have specific biomarkers or are not still capable of identifying the patients that will benefit most from parathyroid surgical therapy.

References

1. Wolf M. Mineral (Mal) adaptation to kidney disease. CJASN. 2015;10(10):1875–85.
2. Martin KJ, González EA. Metabolic bone disease in chronic kidney disease. J Am Soc Nephrol. 2007;18:875–85.
3. McCann LM, Beto J. Roles of calcium-sensing receptor and vitamin D receptor in the pathophysiology of secondary hyperparathyroidism. J Ren Nutr. 2010;20:141–50.
4. Cozzolino M, Mazzaferro S. The fibroblast growth factor 23: a new player in the field of cardiovascular, bone and renal disease. Curr Vasc Pharmacol. 2010;8(3):404–11.
5. Koizumi M, Komaba H, Fukagawa M. Parathyroid function in chronic kidney disease: role of FGF23-Klotho axis. Contrib Nephrol. 2013;180:110–23.

6. Vervloet M. Renal and extrarenal effects of fibroblast growth factor 23. Nat Rev Nephrol. 2019;15:109–20.
7. Kuro-o M. The Klotho proteins in health and disease. Nat Rev Nephrol. 2019;15:27–44.
8. Cozzolino M, Mazzaferro S. Is chronic kidney disease-mineral bone disorder (CKD-MBD) really a syndrome. Nephrol Dial Transpl. 2014;29(10):1815–20.
9. Covic A. Bone and mineral disorders in chronic kidney disease: implications for cardiovascular health and ageing in the general population. Lancet Diabet Endo. 2018;6(4):P319–31.
10. Goto S, Komaba H, Fukagawa M: Pathophysiology of parathyroid hyperplasia in chronic kidney disease: preclinical and clinical basis for parathyroid intervention. NDT Plus. 2008;1(Suppl 3): iii2–8.
11. Cunningham J, Locatelli F. Secondary hyperparathyroidism: Pathogenesis, disease progression, and therapeutic options. Clin J Am Soc Nephrol. 2011;6:913–21.
12. Kidney Disease: Improving Global Outcomes (KDIGO) CKD-MBD Update Work Group. KDIGO. Clinical practice guideline update for the diagnosis, evaluation, prevention, and treatment of Chronic Kidney Disease-Mineral and Bone Disorder (CKD-MBD). Kidney Int Suppl. 2017;2017(7):1–59.
13. Shih ML, Duh QY, Hsieh CB, et al. Total parathyroidectomy without autotransplantation for secondary hyperparathyroidism. World J Surg. 2009;33:248–54. https://doi.org/10.1007/s00268-008-9765-8.
14. Foley RN, Li S. The fall and rise of parathyroidectomy in U.S. hemodialysis patients, 1992 to 2002. J Am Soc Nephrol. 2005;16(1):210–8.
15. National Kidney Foundation. K/DOQI clinical practice guidelines for bone metabolism and disease in chronic kidney disease. Am J Kidney Dis. 2003;42(Suppl 3):S1–202.
16. Kidney Disease: Improving global outcomes CKDMBDWG. KDIGO clinical practice guideline for the diagnosis, evaluation, prevention, and treatment of Chronic Kidney Disease-Mineral and Bone Disorder (CKD-MBD). Kidney Int Suppl. 2009;S1–130.
17. Tentori F, Wang M. Bieber BA recent changes in therapeutic approaches and association with outcomes among patients with secondary hyperparathyroidism on chronic hemodialysis: the DOPPS study. Clin J Am Soc Nephrol. 2015;10:98–109.
18. Wetmore JB. Geographic variation of parathyroidectomy in patients receiving hemodialysis: a retrospective cohort analysis. BMC Surg. 2016;16:77.
19. Kim SM. Rates and outcomes of parathyroidectomy for secondary hyperparathyroidism in the United States. CJASN. 2016;11(7):1260–67.
20. Anderson K Jr. Subtotal versus total parathyroidectomy with autotransplantation for patients with renal hyperparathyroidism have similar outcomes. Am J Surg. 2017;214(5):914–19.
21. Liu ME. To assess the effects of parathyroidectomy (TPTX versus TPTX+AT) for secondary hyperparathyroidism in chronic renal failure: a systematic review and meta-analysis. Int J Surg. 2017;44:353–62.
22. Chen J. Total parathyroidectomy with autotransplantation versus subtotal parathyroidectomy for renal hyperparathyroidism: a systematic review and meta-analysis. Nephrol (Carlton). 2017;22(5):388–96.
23. El-Husseini A. Parathyroidectomy-A last resort for hyperparathyroidism in dialysis patients. Semin Dial. 2017;30(5):385–9.
24. Mazzaferro S, Tartaglione L. Multicenter study on parathyroidectomy (PTX) in Italy: preliminary results. J Nephrol. 2018;31(5):767–73.
25. Mazzaferro S, Pasquali M. Parathyroidectomy as a therapeutic tool for targeting the recommended NKF-K/DOQI ranges for serum calcium, phosphate and parathyroid hormone in dialysis patients. Nephrol Dial Transpl. 2008;23(7):2319–23.
26. Wetmore JB, Liu J. Changes in secondary hyperparathyroidism-related biochemical parameters and medication use following parathyroidectomy. Nephrol Dial Transpl. 2016;31(1):103–11.

27. Kestenbaum B, Andress DL. Survival following parathyroidectomy among United States dialysis patients. Kidney Int. 2004;66(5):2010–6.
28. Ishani A. Clinical outcomes after parathyroidectomy in a nationwide cohort of patients on hemodialysis. CJASN. 2015;10(1):90–7.
29. Ivarsson KM, Akaberi S. The effect of parathyroidectomy on patient survival in secondary hyperparathyroidism. Nephrol Dial Transpl. 2015;30(12):2027–33.
30. Komaba H, Taniguchi M. Parathyroidectomy and survival among Japanese hemodialysis patients with secondary hyperparathyroidism. Kidney Int. 2015;88(2):350–9.
31. Scialla JJ, Wolf M. When there will never be a randomized controlled trial. Kidney Int. 2015;88(2):220–2.
32. Lim CTS. Clinical course after parathyroidectomy in adults with end-stage renal disease on maintenance dialysis. Clin Kidney J. 2018;11(2):265–9.
33. Rudser KD, de Boer IH. Fracture risk after parathyroidectomy among chronic hemodialysis patients. J Am Soc Nephrol. 2007;18(8):2401–7.
34. Isaksson Elin. The effect of parathyroidectomy on risk of hip fracture in secondary hyperparathyroidism. World J Surg. 2017;41(9):2304–11.
35. Lou I. Parathyroidectomy is underutilized in patients with tertiary hyperparathyroidism after renal transplantation. Surgery. 2016;159(1):172–80.
36. Hernandes FR. The shift from high to low turnover bone disease after parathyroidectomy is associated with the progression of vascular calcification in hemodialysis patients: A 12-month follow-up study. PLoS ONE. 12(4):e0174811.

Relation Between PTH and the Risk of Mortality in CKD

Mugurel Apetrii and Adrian Covic

Introduction

Chronic kidney disease (CKD) is highly prevalent and it is associated with a high mortality rate [1]. Several traditional factors like hypertension and diabetes are the most common causes of CKD in the entire world but in the same time they lead to increased cardiovascular mortality. Mortality in patients with CKD, however, can also be attributed to non-traditional risk factors such as inflammation, oxidative stress, anemia, and disorders of the mineral and bone metabolism associated with CKD (CKD-MBD). Secondary hyperparathyroidism (sHPT), a common complication of CKD, is a very important component of the CKD-MBD being characterized by elevated serum parathyroid hormone levels secondary to derangements in the homeostasis of calcium, phosphate, and vitamin D.

Frequently, several-fold higher concentrations of intact parathormone (iPTH) are required to maintain normal bone turnover among patients with end stage renal disease (ESRD), known as skeletal resistance to PTH [2]. This phenomenon is partly due to the diminished PTH receptor expression of osteoblast in the uremic milieu [3]. Also, accumulated truncated 7–84 PTH fragments in patients with ESRD interferes with the type 1 PTH receptor (PTHR1) and with second generation intact PTH assays, resulting in misleadingly higher values of PTH [4]. Therefore, clinicians have to evaluate trends in PTH (and not single values) together with other circulating bone biomarkers like phosphate or total and bone-specific alkaline phosphatases in order to get the whole picture of the CKD-MBD.

A low PTH state could also be a feature of the dysregulated bone and mineral metabolism in CKD. From a morpho-pathological point of view, this condition includes osteomalacia and adynamic bone disease both being associated with low

M. Apetrii (✉) · A. Covic
University of Medicine and Pharmacy "Grigore T. Popa", Iaşi, Romania
e-mail: mugurel.apetrii@gmail.com

© Springer Nature Switzerland AG 2020
A. Covic et al. (eds.), *Parathyroid Glands in Chronic Kidney Disease*,
https://doi.org/10.1007/978-3-030-43769-5_13

187

bone turnover leading to poor mineralization. The incidence of adynamic bone disease increasing is partially secondary to PTH over-suppression from calcium overload, vitamin D agents, calcimimetics, and phosphate binders [5].

Parathormone and Mortality in the General Population

The prevalence of hypertension among individuals with primary hyperparathyroidism ranges from 30 to 70%, and blood pressure decreases following surgical parathyroidectomy (PTX) [6, 7]. Furthermore, in patients with normal renal function, higher serum iPTH concentrations are known to be associated with coronary artery disease, increased left ventricular mass [8], and heart failure [9]. A possible causal link between cardiovascular disease and PTH may be represented by the stimulatory actions of PTH upon the renin–angiotensin–aldosterone system leading to increased levels of angiotensin II and aldosterone, which in turn cause left ventricular remodelling and arterial hypertension [10]. Although, the proof of a causal role for PTH in cardiovascular disease is still lacking, several underlying mechanisms that might explain this association have been proposed. Thus, PTH could induce direct detrimental myocardial effects favouring cardiac ischaemia or an increased risk for heart failure of non-ischaemic origin. Secondly, PTH excess has been linked with arterial stiffness and hypertension increased PTH that may induce endothelial dysfunction and atherosclerosis. And finally, data from a meta-analysis of PTX effects upon left ventricular hypertrophy (LVH) support the hypothesis of a causal link between PTH and LVH since LVH regressed in most patients with primary HPT after surgery [11].

Only few observational data suggests that higher levels of PTH in patients with normal renal function are associated with death from cardiovascular disease [9, 12]. although other have failed to demonstrate this link [13]. Therefore, giving the observational nature of these studies and the discordant results, we cannot postulate that PTH excess plays a causal role in the development of cardiovascular disease since this serologic marker might be only an indicator of health status.

Parathormone and Mortality in CKD

Cardiovascular disease is one of the main complication associated with either low of high PTH in CKD patients, due to the major 'off-target' effects of PTH in the cardiovascular system. The derangements in calcium and phosphate that result from sHPT may accelerate vascular calcifications, including coronary artery calcification therefore increasing the risk of death. Medial calcification is one of the complication of longstanding severe sHPT and is classically associated with high serum levels of calcium and phosphate. When it touches the arterioles of the skin and soft tissue it could lead to necrosis or ulceration, a condition known as calcific uremic arteriolopathy or calciphylaxis, being associated with an eight-fold increase in mortality rate [14].

Numerous cohort studies reported significant and independent associations between serum PTH levels and adverse outcomes including mortality in CKD patients. Importantly, this association is usually J-shaped, suggesting an 'optimal PTH' range for these specific outcomes, which could be ~150–300 pg/mL in dialysis patients [15]. Kalantar-Zadeh et al. in a large cohort of haemodialysis patients showed that, high levels of PTH were associated with increased risk of death [16]. Thus, using time-dependent models, the authors showed that PTH levels between 300 and 600 pg/ml were incrementally associated with higher death risk when compared to the 150 to 300 pg/ml for the reference group.

In a secondary analysis of the SPRINT trial, the participants with CKD and higher PTH had a greater associated risk of cardiovascular events and received less cardiovascular protection from intensive blood pressure therapy than participants with a lower serum PTH [17]. Moreover, there was no evidence that fibroblast growth factor 23 (FGF23) concentrations modified the relationship of intensive blood pressure lowering with higher PTH levels.

In observational studies of patients with end-stage renal disease, serum PTH levels have exhibited either a positively association with mortality, [18, 19] an U-shaped association [20] or no association with mortality [21]. These inconsistent findings may be explained by unmeasured or residual confounding by their residual kidney function. Thus, in a large cohort of incident haemodialysis patients, higher iPTH levels were associated with lower mortality among patients on hemodialysis with low residual renal function, whereas higher iPTH levels showed a higher mortality risk among patients with substantial renal kidney function [22]. Mortality risk in patients with preserved residual renal function was also higher in those with high phosphate, even if residual kidney function contributes to substantial clearance of phosphorus in patients with ESRD. Higher mortality risk associates with high iPTH and phosphate may therefore indicate nonadherence to diet, haemodialysis prescription, and/or medications, including phosphate binders and cinacalcet [22]. Furthermore, this association between serum PTH levels and mortality differs according to the level of residual kidney function [22]. In incident dialysis patients, the impact of the delta iPTH during the first year of dialysis on mortality shows also a J-shaped form. A mild increase (<300 pg/ml) appears to be associated with lower mortality, although this association was not significant in patients with higher delta iPTH. Conversely, low iPTH mostly induced by high dialysate calcium appears as an independent risk factor for cardiovascular death in these patients.

The Effect of PTH Lowering Therapies on Mortality

Assuming that PTH is a uremic toxin and associated with poor survival in CKD, as shown by Kovesdy et al. [23] normalization of serum PTH levels using either vitamin D, phosphate binders, calcimimetics or even PTX might be an attractive option for the clinicians. However, studies trying to see if the drugs used widely in CKD to correct perturbed serum PTH correlate with cardiovascular and all-cause mortality revealed more discrepant results. Although the effects of these drugs in standard clinical practice are universally measured based on improvements in levels of such biomarkers, a recent meta-analysis of Palmer et al. of randomized trials failed to see such a correlation [24]. This seems more disturbing since in general, these drugs showed large effects on reducing PTH, but effects on mortality outcomes were much smaller and generally not statistically significant. These results were confirmed by another large randomized trial (the EVOLVE study) and a meta-analysis both showing no effect on mortality of cinacalcet, a well-known calcimimetic drug which efficiently decreases serum PTH levels [25, 26]. A secondary analysis, however, found an approximately 12% reduction in the composite endpoint when adjusted for a variety of demographic and clinical factors. Although the predefined secondary and post hoc analyses of the EVOLVE trial suggested beneficial effects both in general and in subgroups, it has been proposed that cinacalcet should be used to improve the achievement of biochemical control of CKD-MBD and not with the purpose of reducing cardiovascular outcomes and/or improving survival [27].

These discordant results between biochemical endpoints and mortality endpoint are not new in the field of nephrology, similar to erythropoietin treatment, hemoglobin level and mortality or statins, cholesterol level and mortality in dialyzed patients [27–29]. Therefore, caution is needed before accepting biochemical outcomes as relevant to drug research.

Besides some methodological issues (e.g. small number of patients, short period of follow-up for some studies) that could explain the lack of association between PTH lowering drugs and hard endpoints, there are some other issues that had to be considered. First, even if these medications by lowering PTH and normalizing the other CKD-MBD parameters interfere with causal pathways of vascular calcification and injury, the pathologic mechanisms causing death in these patients are poorly understood. One possibility is that other biological pathways are more relevant to health outcomes in CKD patients and maybe the drugs used for bone disease may only partially modify some pathophysiologic pathways causing cardiovascular disease that are mediated through the biochemical markers and vascular calcifications. However, even if existing evidence suggests a lack of effect of these drugs on mortality, other outcomes influenced by these medications might be significant for the patient. Thus, ameliorating itching, fracture incidence, bone pain, muscle weakness, impaired physical function, and quality of life may be some of the beneficial effects of these medications interfering with CKD-MBD parameters and should be properly evaluated in future clinical trials to establish if they are relevant to clinical practice.

Furthermore, a recent metanalysis including almost 25,000 patients suggests suggest a clinically significant beneficial effect of PTX on all-cause and cardiovascular mortality in CKD patients with sHPT [30]. This improvement of outcome might be related to the amelioration of hypertension [31] and the attenuation of cardiac hypertrophy via a decreased FGF23 level after PTX [32]. In addition to this, the coronary artery calcification is also alleviated or stable after PTX via an increased post PTX Fetuin-A level, a known inhibitor of extra osseous calcification [33, 34]. However, this analysis comprises only observational studies being therefore subject to bias and considerable heterogeneity. Nevertheless, as compared to medication, PTX significantly improved not only the biochemical endpoints but more importantly it decreased the all-cause mortality by almost 30 percent, a proper-conducted randomized controlled trial to compare parathyroidectomy with non-surgical therapy for sHPT associated with CKD is needed in order to validate these results.

References

1. Hill NR, Fatoba ST, Oke JL, Hirst JA, O'Callaghan CA, Lasserson DS, et al. Global prevalence of chronic kidney disease—a systematic review and meta-analysis. PLoS One. 2016;11(7):e0158765.
2. Iwasaki Y, Yamato H, Nii-Kono T, Fujieda A, Uchida M, Hosokawa A, et al. Insufficiency of PTH action on bone in uremia. Kidney Int Suppl. 2006;102:S34–6.
3. Nii-Kono T, Iwasaki Y, Uchida M, Fujieda A, Hosokawa A, Motojima M, et al. Indoxyl sulfate induces skeletal resistance to parathyroid hormone in cultured osteoblastic cells. Kidney Int. 2007;71(8):738–43.
4. Slatopolsky E, Finch J, Clay P, Martin D, Sicard G, Singer G, et al. A novel mechanism for skeletal resistance in uremia. Kidney Int. 2000;58(2):753–61.
5. Andress DL. Adynamic bone in patients with chronic kidney disease. Kidney Int. 2008;73(12):1345–54.
6. Kalla A, Krishnamoorthy P, Gopalakrishnan A, Garg J, Patel NC, Figueredo VM. Primary hyperparathyroidism predicts hypertension: Results from the national inpatient sample. Int J Cardiol. 2017;227:335–7.
7. Sofronie AC, Kooij I, Bursot C, Santagati G, Coindre JP, Piccoli GB. Full normalization of severe hypertension after parathryoidectomy—a case report and systematic review. BMC Nephrol. 2018;19(1):112.
8. Saleh FN, Schirmer H, Sundsfjord J, Jorde R. Parathyroid hormone and left ventricular hypertrophy. Eur Heart J. 2003;24(22):2054–60.
9. Kestenbaum B, Katz R, de Boer I, Hoofnagle A, Sarnak MJ, Shlipak MG, et al. Vitamin D, parathyroid hormone, and cardiovascular events among older adults. J Am Coll Cardiol. 2011;58(14):1433–41.
10. Vaidya A, Brown JM, Williams JS. The renin-angiotensin-aldosterone system and calcium-regulatory hormones. J Hum Hypertens. 2015;29(9):515–21.
11. Donald J. McMahon, Angela Carrelli, Nick Palmeri, Chiyuan Zhang, Marco DiTullio, Shonni J. Silverberg, Marcella D. Walker, (2015) Effect of Parathyroidectomy Upon Left Ventricular Mass in Primary Hyperparathyroidism: A Meta-Analysis. The Journal of Clinical Endocrinology & Metabolism 100 (12):4399-4407
12. Hagstrom E, Hellman P, Larsson TE, Ingelsson E, Berglund L, Sundstrom J, et al. Plasma parathyroid hormone and the risk of cardiovascular mortality in the community. Circulation. 2009;119(21):2765–71.
13. Reid LJ, Muthukrishnan B, Patel D, Seckl JR, Gibb FW. Predictors of nephrolithiasis, osteoporosis and mortality in primary hyperparathyroidism. J Clin Endocrinol Metab. 2019.
14. Mazhar AR, Johnson RJ, Gillen D, Stivelman JC, Ryan MJ, Davis CL, et al. Risk factors and mortality associated with calciphylaxis in end-stage renal disease. Kidney Int. 2001;60(1):324–32.
15. Lau WL, Kalantar-Zadeh K, Kovesdy CP, Mehrotra R. Alkaline phosphatase: better than PTH as a marker of cardiovascular and bone disease? Hemodial Int Int Sympos Home Hemodial. 2014;18(4):720–4.

16. Kalantar-Zadeh K, Kuwae N, Regidor DL, Kovesdy CP, Kilpatrick RD, Shinaberger CS, et al. Survival predictability of time-varying indicators of bone disease in maintenance hemodialysis patients. Kidney Int. 2006;70(4):771–80.

17. Ginsberg C, Craven TE, Chonchol MB, Cheung AK, Sarnak MJ, Ambrosius WT, et al. PTH, FGF23, and intensive blood pressure lowering in chronic kidney disease participants in SPRINT. Clin J Am Soc Nephrol. 2018;13(12):1816–24.

18. Slinin Y, Foley RN, Collins AJ. Calcium, phosphorus, parathyroid hormone, and cardiovascular disease in hemodialysis patients: the USRDS waves 1, 3, and 4 study. J Am Soc Nephrol. 2005;16(6):1788–93.

19. Young EW, Albert JM, Satayathum S, Goodkin DA, Pisoni RL, Akiba T, et al. Predictors and consequences of altered mineral metabolism: the dialysis outcomes and practice patterns study. Kidney Int. 2005;67(3):1179–87.

20. Floege J, Kim J, Ireland E, Chazot C, Drueke T, de Francisco A, et al. Serum iPTH, calcium and phosphate, and the risk of mortality in a European haemodialysis population. Nephrol Dial Transplant. 2011;26(6):1948–55.

21. Liu CT, Lin YC, Lin YC, Kao CC, Chen HH, Hsu CC, et al. Roles of serum Calcium, Phosphorus, PTH and ALP on mortality in peritoneal dialysis patients: A nationwide, population-based longitudinal study using TWRDS 2005–2012. Sci Rep. 2017;7(1):33.

22. Wang M, Obi Y, Streja E, Rhee CM, Lau WL, Chen J, et al. Association of parameters of mineral bone disorder with mortality in patients on hemodialysis according to level of residual kidney function. Clin J Am Soc Nephrol. 2017;12(7):1118–27.

23. Kovesdy CP, Ahmadzadeh S, Anderson JE, Kalantar-Zadeh K. Secondary hyperparathyroidism is associated with higher mortality in men with moderate to severe chronic kidney disease. Kidney Int. 2008;73(11):1296–302.

24. Palmer SC, Teixeira-Pinto A, Saglimbene V, Craig JC, Macaskill P, Tonelli M, et al. Association of drug effects on serum parathyroid Hormone, Phosphorus, and Calcium levels with mortality in CKD: A meta-analysis. Am J Kidney Dis. 2015;66(6):962–71.

25. Chertow GM, Block GA, Correa-Rotter R, Drueke TB, Floege J, Goodman WG, et al. Effect of cinacalcet on cardiovascular disease in patients undergoing dialysis. N Engl J Med. 2012;367(26):2482–94.

26. Palmer SC, Nistor I, Craig JC, Pellegrini F, Messa P, Tonelli M, et al. Cinacalcet in patients with chronic kidney disease: a cumulative meta-analysis of randomized controlled trials. PLoS Med. 2013;10(4):e1001436.

27. Goldsmith D, Covic A, Vervloet M, Cozzolino M, Nistor I. Should patients with CKD stage 5D and biochemical evidence of secondary hyperparathyroidism be prescribed calcimimetic therapy? An ERA-EDTA position statement. Nephrol Dial Transplant. 2015;30(5):698–700.

28. Phrommintikul A, Haas SJ, Elsik M, Krum H. Mortality and target haemoglobin concentrations in anaemic patients with chronic kidney disease treated with erythropoietin: a meta-analysis. Lancet. 2007;369(9559):381–8.

29. Fellstrom BC, Jardine AG, Schmieder RE, Holdaas H, Bannister K, Beutler J, et al. Rosuvastatin and cardiovascular events in patients undergoing hemodialysis. N Engl J Med. 2009;360(14):1395–407.

30. Apetrii M, Goldsmith D, Nistor I, Siriopol D, Voroneanu L, Scripcariu D, et al. Impact of surgical parathyroidectomy on chronic kidney disease-mineral and bone disorder (CKD-MBD)—a systematic review and meta-analysis. PLoS One. 2017;12(11):e0187025.

31. Goldsmith DJ, Covic AA, Venning MC, Ackrill P. Blood pressure reduction after parathyroidectomy for secondary hyperparathyroidism: further evidence implicating calcium homeostasis in blood pressure regulation. Am J Kidney Dis. 1996;27(6):819–25.

32. Takahashi H, Komaba H, Takahashi Y, Sawada K, Tatsumi R, Kanai G, et al. Impact of parathyroidectomy on serum FGF23 and soluble Klotho in hemodialysis patients with severe secondary hyperparathyroidism. J Clin Endocrinol Metab. 2014;99(4):E652–8.

33. Bleyer AJ, Burkart J, Piazza M, Russell G, Rohr M, Carr JJ. Changes in cardiovascular calcification after parathyroidectomy in patients with ESRD. Am J Kidney Dis. 2005;46(3):464–9.
34. Wang CC, Hsu YJ, Wu CC, Yang SS, Chen GS, Lin SH, et al. Serum fetuin-A levels increased following parathyroidectomy in uremic hyperparathyroidism. Clin Nephrol. 2012;77(2):89–96.

Index

© Springer Nature Switzerland AG 2020
A. Covic et al. (eds.), *Parathyroid Glands in Chronic Kidney Disease*,
https://doi.org/10.1007/978-3-030-43769-5

Printed in the United States
by Baker & Taylor Publisher Services